Conquering Chiari

A Care Guide

BELINDA SNOW

DEDICATION

To Pat, whose strength and courage inspire us all. Your journey through Chiari Malformation, with grace and resilience, has touched the hearts of many. This book is dedicated to you and all the brave individuals facing similar challenges, with the hope that it brings greater understanding and awareness.

— Belinda Snow

Contents

Introduction...1

1 What is Chiari Malformation?................................5

2 Types of Chiari...11

3 Getting a Diagnosis...17

4 Differential Diagnoses...23

5 Treatment Options...29

6 Outcomes 35

7 Recovery 41

8 Living with Chiari..47

9 Workplace and Educational Challenges 59

10 Mental Health 67

11. Controversies in Chiari 73

12 Current Research into Chiari 79

13 Looking Ahead...85

14. FAQ..89

14. Beware of Quackery 95

Glossary for Medical and Technical Terms.............102

Appendix: Resources and Support...........................109

References 115

About the Author 117

Chiari Malformation is a complex neurological disorder that affects thousands of individuals worldwide. Despite its growing recognition, for many, the journey to a diagnosis can be long and fraught with confusion, misdiagnosis, and frustration. Chiari Malformation often presents with a wide range of symptoms that are easily attributed to other conditions, leaving many patients in search of answers for years. The diagnosis itself can feel overwhelming, triggering a flood of questions and uncertainties about the future—what treatments are available, what lifestyle changes might be necessary, and how to cope with the emotional and physical toll. This book, *Conquering Chiari*, is designed to be a comprehensive, clear, and compassionate guide for patients, families, and caregivers navigating the challenges of this condition.

Understanding Chiari Malformation can be daunting, especially when the medical terminology is unfamiliar and the path forward is unclear. The goal of this book is to bridge the gap between the clinical world and the everyday experiences of those living with Chiari Malformation. Whether you are someone newly diagnosed, a parent grappling with what this diagnosis means for your child, or a patient in the midst of treatment or recovery, this book provides not only medical insights but also practical advice and emotional support.

Chiari Malformation Type I (CM-1) is the most common

form of this condition, characterized by the downward displacement of the cerebellar tonsils—a portion of the brain—into the spinal canal. This displacement can disrupt the normal flow of cerebrospinal fluid (CSF), leading to a variety of symptoms that may include debilitating headaches, balance problems, neck pain, and even more severe neurological deficits. The severity of symptoms varies widely from person to person: some individuals may go years without noticeable issues, while others experience life-altering symptoms that significantly reduce their quality of life. For this reason, early diagnosis and proper management are critical to preventing further complications and improving outcomes. However, despite advances in diagnostic imaging, particularly the use of magnetic resonance imaging (MRI), many patients still face a prolonged diagnostic process that can leave them feeling helpless and uncertain about their future.

The increasing awareness of Chiari Malformation has brought to light the need for accessible, reliable resources for those affected by the condition. A diagnosis of CM often raises more questions than answers: What does it mean for long-term health? Will surgery be required, and what are the risks? How can I manage daily symptoms? This book seeks to address those questions by providing up-to-date information that explains the complexities of Chiari Malformation in a way that is easy to understand. It also includes guidance on navigating the healthcare system, from finding the right specialists to understanding treatment options, and offers advice on how to advocate for yourself or a loved one.

My inspiration to write this book comes from a deeply personal experience. A close friend's daughter was diagnosed with Chiari Malformation at a young age, and watching their family's struggle to get the right diagnosis and treatment was both heart-wrenching and eye-opening. The road to understanding the condition and finding the right medical care was long and confusing, marked by moments of fear and uncertainty. I witnessed firsthand the emotional and physical toll this diagnosis took on the family—the stress of managing a chronic illness, the challenges of navigating a medical system that often felt indifferent, and the emotional weight of seeing a loved one in pain. These experiences inspired me to use my background in health sciences and education to create a resource that could provide the kind of support my friend's family needed during their journey.

With more than 30 years of experience writing about health sciences, I've come to appreciate how important it is for patients and families to have clear, accurate, and actionable information at their fingertips. This book was written with that goal in mind. While there is an abundance of medical literature available, much of it can feel inaccessible to the average person. My aim is to translate complex medical concepts into practical advice, empowering readers to take an active role in their healthcare journey.

One of the key themes in *Conquering Chiari* is the importance of becoming an informed advocate for yourself or your loved one. Chiari Malformation is a lifelong condition that requires ongoing management, and having the knowledge to ask the right questions and make informed decisions is essential. This book is structured to guide you through the stages of understanding your diagnosis, exploring treatment options, and preparing for possible surgery. Each chapter is dedicated to addressing the most critical aspects of life with Chiari Malformation: from the day-to-day management of symptoms to navigating the healthcare system, to the emotional and psychological impacts of living with a chronic illness. By demystifying the condition and providing concrete steps to take, this book equips you with the tools to advocate for the best care possible.

For many, the decision to undergo surgery is one of the most difficult aspects of living with Chiari Malformation. The procedure most commonly recommended is suboccipital decompression, which aims to relieve the pressure caused by the herniated cerebellar tonsils and restore the normal flow of cerebrospinal fluid. While surgery can offer significant relief, it is not a cure, and the outcomes can vary. In some cases, symptoms may persist or recur after surgery, making post-operative care and monitoring crucial. In *Conquering Chiari Malformation*, I explain the surgical process in detail, outlining what to expect before, during, and after surgery, as well as the potential risks and benefits. I also provide real-life accounts from patients who have undergone surgery, offering their insights on recovery and long-term management.

Beyond the physical aspects of the condition, *Conquering Chiari* also addresses the emotional and mental health challenges that often accompany a diagnosis. Living with a chronic illness like CM can lead to feelings of isolation, anxiety, and depression. The uncertainty of the future, the pain and discomfort of symptoms, and the disruption of daily life can take a heavy toll on emotional well-being. This book offers strategies for coping with the psychological impact of CM, emphasizing the importance of seeking professional mental health support and building a strong support network of family, friends, and healthcare providers.

In addition to providing medical information and coping strategies, *Conquering Chiari* includes real-life stories from patients and families who have walked the same path. These stories illustrate the wide range of experiences people with CM face, from the frustration of misdiagnosis to the relief of finally finding the right treatment. These personal accounts highlight the resilience and determination that is often required to live with Chiari Malformation and offer hope to those who may be struggling to see a way forward.

The goal of *Conquering Chiari* is not just to inform but to inspire. I want this book to serve as a source of knowledge and empowerment for anyone affected by Chiari Malformation. Whether you are a patient, a parent, or a caregiver, my hope is that this book provides you with the tools you need to navigate the challenges ahead with confidence and courage.

By offering expert insights, personal stories, and practical advice, *Conquering Chiari* serves as both a guide and a companion on your journey toward understanding, managing, and ultimately conquering Chiari Malformation.

1 What is Chiari Malformation?

Chiari Malformation (CM) is a structural defect in the brain that affects the space where the brain and spinal cord meet. It occurs when the lower part of the brain, known as the cerebellum, descends out of its normal position and extends into the spinal canal. This displacement can compress the brainstem and disrupt the flow of cerebrospinal fluid (CSF), the liquid that surrounds and protects the brain and spinal cord.

In a healthy person, the cerebellum sits comfortably within the base of the skull, in an area known as the posterior fossa. When this part of the brain slips downward, as in Chiari malformation, it can lead to a host of neurological symptoms, ranging from mild discomfort to debilitating pain and loss of function.

There are several types of Chiari malformation, but the most common form is **Chiari Type I**, which is often diagnosed in late childhood or adulthood. Other types, such as Chiari Type II and Chiari Type III, are typically more severe and are often diagnosed in infancy.

Common Symptoms of Chiari Malformation

One of the most challenging aspects of Chiari malformation is its wide range of symptoms. Some individuals with CM may have few or no symptoms, while others may experience severe and life-altering effects. Symptoms are often related to the compression of the brainstem, cerebellum, or spinal cord and the disruption of CSF flow.

Some of the most common symptoms include:

- **Headaches**: Often at the back of the head, these headaches are typically brought on or exacerbated by physical activities such as coughing, sneezing, or straining.

- **Neck pain**: Chronic pain in the neck area, often radiating down the shoulders.

- **Balance problems**: Dizziness, clumsiness, and unsteadiness are common as the cerebellum, which controls balance and coordination, is compressed.

- **Muscle weakness**: This may manifest in the arms, legs, or other areas of the body.

- **Tingling or numbness**: Many people with CM experience abnormal sensations, especially in the hands and feet.

- **Difficulty swallowing**: Known as dysphagia, some patients struggle with swallowing due to brainstem compression, which controls basic functions like swallowing and breathing.

- **Ringing in the ears** (tinnitus): A high-pitched ringing or buzzing in the ears can occur due to nerve compression.

- **Vision problems**: Blurred or double vision is not uncommon.

- **Sleep apnea**: Some individuals with CM experience interrupted breathing during sleep.

- **Fatigue**: Chronic tiredness and a general feeling of being unwell often accompany Chiari malformation.

Related Conditions

Chiari malformation is often associated with other neurological and spinal conditions, some of which can complicate the diagnosis and treatment process. These related conditions include:

1.   **Syringomyelia**: A condition in which a fluid-filled cyst, or syrinx, forms within the spinal cord. Syringomyelia is common in individuals with Chiari malformation because the abnormal flow of CSF can lead to the development of the syrinx, which compresses the spinal cord and causes pain, weakness, and other symptoms.

2.   **Hydrocephalus**: This is the buildup of excess CSF in the brain's ventricles, leading to increased pressure on the brain. Hydrocephalus can develop in some individuals with Chiari malformation due to the abnormal flow of CSF.

3.   **Ehlers-Danlos Syndrome (EDS)**: This genetic disorder affects connective tissue, leading to joint hypermobility, fragile skin, and blood vessel problems. There is a notable association between Chiari malformation and EDS, particularly because individuals with EDS may have looser connective tissues in the spinal region, which can exacerbate the downward herniation of the cerebellum.

4.   **Tethered Cord Syndrome**: This occurs when the spinal cord becomes attached to tissues inside the spine, causing abnormal stretching and tension. It is often found in individuals with Chiari malformation, and the symptoms of tethered cord can mimic or worsen those of Chiari.

5.   **Scoliosis**: Abnormal curvature of the spine is sometimes seen in individuals with Chiari malformation, particularly if they also have syringomyelia.

6.   **Spina Bifida**: Chiari malformation Type II is strongly associated with spina bifida, a birth defect

where the spinal cord doesn't develop properly. This form of Chiari is typically diagnosed in infancy or early childhood and involves more severe neurological impairments.

A Personal Story: Pat's Journey with Chiari Malformation

Pat was a vibrant and curious child when she first began experiencing symptoms that no one in her family could explain. What started as occasional headaches soon escalated to severe pain that would leave her in tears. At times, she would become dizzy and fall, losing her balance without warning. Even her vision was affected; there were days when everything seemed to blur, and she struggled to focus in school.

Her parents initially thought it was just growing pains or stress from her busy school life, but as the symptoms worsened, they knew something more serious was going on. After multiple visits to different doctors, Pat was referred to a neurologist who, after an MRI scan, delivered the diagnosis: Chiari malformation Type I.

For Pat, the news was both a relief and a source of fear. Finally, there was an explanation for her suffering, but the idea that her brain was pressing into her spinal canal was terrifying. She and her family quickly realized that Chiari malformation wasn't just a condition with a simple fix. It required careful management, and for some patients, surgery might be necessary to relieve the pressure on the brain and spinal cord.

As a young child, Pat had to navigate a world where her peers didn't understand her condition. On bad days, the headaches would force her to stay home from school, and on good days, she was still limited in how much she could physically exert herself. Activities like running or even laughing too hard could trigger severe pain.

Pat's journey with Chiari malformation wasn't straightforward. While she was initially managed with medication to control the pain and physical therapy to help with balance issues, her symptoms eventually worsened. By the time she was in her teens, she faced the decision of whether to undergo decompression surgery—a procedure that would remove a small portion of the bone at the back of her skull to create more space for the brain and improve CSF flow.

The decision wasn't easy. Surgery came with risks, but without it, Pat's quality of life would continue to decline. With the support of her family and her doctors, she opted for surgery, hoping it would alleviate the constant pressure and pain that had come to dominate her life.

Thankfully, Pat's surgery was successful. While recovery was long and challenging, she emerged from it with a significant reduction in her symptoms. She still experiences occasional headaches and balance issues, but the improvement in her daily life has been substantial.

Pat's story is just one example of the many challenges faced by those with Chiari malformation. Each patient's experience is unique, and while some individuals may manage their symptoms with conservative treatments, others, like Pat, may require more invasive interventions.

The Importance of Early Detection

One of the most critical aspects of managing Chiari malformation is early detection. Because the symptoms can be so varied and sometimes vague, many individuals go undiagnosed for years. In some cases, a diagnosis may not occur until adulthood, even though symptoms began in childhood.

For children like Pat, early diagnosis allowed her to receive the care and monitoring she needed. Parents and caregivers should be aware of the common signs of Chiari malformation in children, which can include:

- Chronic headaches, particularly at the base of the skull.

- Difficulty with balance and coordination.

- Weakness or numbness in the arms or legs.

- Developmental delays or issues with fine motor skills.

- Persistent neck pain or stiffness.

- Dizziness or lightheadedness.

- Difficulty swallowing or choking on food.

If any of these symptoms are present, particularly in combination, it's important to consult with a healthcare provider for further evaluation.

Conclusion

Chiari malformation is a complex neurological condition that can significantly impact an individual's quality of life. For children like Pat, early diagnosis and treatment can make a world of difference in managing symptoms and preventing long-term complications. While there is no cure for Chiari malformation, advancements in medical care—ranging from pain management to surgical interventions—offer hope to those living with this challenging condition.

Chiari Malformation (CM) is a structural abnormality at the base of the skull and brain that can affect the brainstem, cerebellum, and spinal cord. This condition results from the cerebellum being pushed down into the spinal canal, disrupting the flow of cerebrospinal fluid (CSF). Chiari Malformations are classified into four types based on the severity of the herniation and the structures involved. Each type varies significantly in terms of symptoms, age of onset, and the extent of the malformation.

1. Type I Chiari Malformation (CM-1)

Type I (CM-1) is the most common form of Chiari Malformation and is often diagnosed in adulthood, although it can be detected in children and adolescents. CM-1 occurs when the cerebellar tonsils—the lower part of the cerebellum—extend into the upper spinal canal through the foramen magnum, the large opening at the base of the skull. In a normal brain, the cerebellar tonsils rest just above the foramen magnum, but in CM-1, these tonsils descend into the spinal canal, potentially leading to a range of neurological symptoms.

Symptoms of CM-1: Many individuals with CM-1 may not experience symptoms, and the malformation may only be discovered incidentally during an MRI scan for another issue. However, in symptomatic cases, CM-1 can cause headaches (especially when coughing, sneezing, or straining), neck pain, dizziness, balance problems, numbness or tingling in the extremities, and difficulties with coordination. In more severe cases, patients may experience neurological symptoms such as weakness, difficulty swallowing, or vision disturbances. Syringomyelia, a condition in which a fluid-filled cyst (syrinx) forms within the spinal cord, can also develop, leading to more serious complications like muscle weakness or paralysis.

Severity and Treatment: The severity of CM-1 varies depending on how much the cerebellar tonsils herniate into the spinal canal and whether it impedes the flow of CSF. Treatment is often based on the severity of symptoms, ranging from monitoring and pain management to surgical intervention (usually a decompression surgery) to alleviate pressure on the brainstem and restore normal CSF flow.

2. Type II Chiari Malformation (CM-2, or Arnold-Chiari Malformation)

Type II Chiari Malformation is more severe than CM-1 and usually diagnosed at birth or in early infancy. In CM-2, both the cerebellum and brainstem herniate into the spinal canal. This form of Chiari Malformation is almost always associated with spina bifida, a birth defect where the spinal cord does not develop properly, leaving part of it exposed.

Symptoms of CM-2: Because CM-2 typically develops during fetal development and is present at birth, its symptoms often manifest early in life. Infants with CM-2 may experience breathing difficulties, trouble swallowing, poor feeding, gagging, vomiting, arm weakness, and developmental delays. The malformation can also cause hydrocephalus (a buildup of fluid in the brain), which may require a shunt to drain the excess fluid. Children with CM-2 are also more likely to develop syringomyelia.

Why is CM-2 More Severe? CM-2 is considered more severe than CM-1 because it involves the downward displacement of both the cerebellum and brainstem, structures that are crucial for vital functions such as breathing, swallowing, and motor control. The herniation of the brainstem into the spinal canal disrupts these critical functions and can lead to life-threatening complications. Additionally, the presence of spina bifida in most CM-2 cases complicates the condition, as it exposes the spinal cord to further damage, increasing the risk of paralysis or other serious neurological impairments.

Treatment for CM-2: Treatment for CM-2 often involves managing the symptoms through surgery. A common procedure is decompression surgery, which aims to increase the space at the base of the skull, allowing the brainstem and cerebellum to return to their normal positions. Shunt placement for hydrocephalus is another frequent intervention. Early diagnosis and treatment are crucial in preventing or mitigating long-term neurological damage.

3. Type III Chiari Malformation (CM-3)

Type III Chiari Malformation is one of the rarest and most severe forms of Chiari Malformation. In CM-3, there is a significant herniation of the cerebellum, brainstem, and sometimes other parts of the brain through an abnormal opening in the back of the skull. This type of malformation is often accompanied by a condition called encephalocele, where parts of the brain protrude through the skull, and there may also be associated spinal defects.

Symptoms of CM-3: Due to the severity of the malformation, infants born with CM-3 usually exhibit profound neurological deficits, which can include severe intellectual disabilities, seizures, muscle weakness, difficulty swallowing, and abnormal breathing patterns. These infants often have hydrocephalus, spina bifida, and other serious developmental issues.

Why is CM-3 More Severe? CM-3 is more severe than CM-1 and CM-2 because it involves more extensive structural abnormalities, including defects in the bones of the skull and spine. The brain's descent through the skull opening is more pronounced, putting significant pressure on the brainstem and cerebellum. This pressure impairs vital brain functions such as regulating breathing, heart rate, and coordination. The malformation often causes severe neurological impairment that can be life-threatening in infancy. The presence of encephalocele further complicates the condition, as it involves a protrusion of brain tissue outside the skull, making it highly susceptible to damage.

Treatment for CM-3: Treatment options for CM-3 are limited and focused on reducing the pressure on the brain and spinal cord and managing the symptoms. Surgery is often necessary to correct the herniation and close any skull or spinal defects. However, due to the complexity and severity of the malformation, the prognosis is often poor, with many infants not surviving beyond early childhood or experiencing significant lifelong disabilities.

4. Type IV Chiari Malformation (CM-4)

Type IV Chiari Malformation is the rarest and most severe form of Chiari Malformation. Unlike the other types, CM-4 is characterized by the underdevelopment or absence of the cerebellum, a part of the brain responsible for coordinating movement and balance. This condition, known as cerebellar hypoplasia or aplasia, leads to profound developmental issues and severe neurological impairment.

Symptoms of CM-4: Children born with CM-4 often exhibit extreme developmental delays, muscle weakness, poor motor coordination, and difficulties with basic functions such as breathing, swallowing, and movement. Many infants with CM-4 do not survive beyond infancy due to the severity of the condition and the involvement of vital brain structures.

Why is CM-4 the Most Severe? CM-4 is the most severe type of Chiari Malformation because it involves not just the displacement of the cerebellum, but its underdevelopment or complete absence. The cerebellum plays a critical role in coordinating motor activities, and without its proper function, essential processes like balance, movement, and reflexes are severely compromised. Infants with CM-4 often have other serious brain malformations, further complicating the prognosis.

Treatment for CM-4: There is no cure for CM-4, and treatment is primarily supportive. Efforts are focused on managing symptoms and improving the infant's quality of life for as long as possible. Palliative care may be necessary to address feeding difficulties, respiratory issues, and other life-threatening complications.

Conclusion: Understanding the Spectrum of Chiari Malformations

Chiari Malformations represent a spectrum of neurological disorders that range from relatively mild in Type I to extremely severe in Types III and IV. Each type presents its own unique challenges in terms of diagnosis, symptoms, and treatment. While CM-1 may often be managed with monitoring or surgery, the more severe forms, such as CM-2, CM-3, and CM-4, can involve significant neurological impairments and require intensive medical intervention. Understanding the differences between these types helps both medical professionals and families make informed decisions about treatment and care.

3 Getting a Diagnosis

Chiari Malformation is a complex condition that often takes years to diagnose due to its wide-ranging and sometimes subtle symptoms. Each patient's journey to diagnosis is unique, and for some, like Pat, it can begin with an unexpected symptom that spirals into a long process of medical testing, consultations, and uncertainty. In this chapter, we explore the various paths that lead to a Chiari diagnosis, the diagnostic tests involved, and the challenges of communicating this diagnosis to others, especially when the symptoms are difficult to explain.

The Elusive Nature of Diagnosis

Chiari Malformation is often referred to as an "invisible condition" because its symptoms can mimic those of many other disorders, making it difficult for both patients and healthcare providers to pinpoint the cause. In fact, many people live with Chiari for years before receiving an accurate diagnosis, especially when their symptoms are mild or intermittent.

Pat's journey to diagnosis began when she was just eight years old. She had always been a quiet child, but she started to complain about frequent headaches and neck pain. Initially, her parents attributed it to normal childhood issues—perhaps stress from school or growing pains. It wasn't until the symptoms became more intense, with occasional dizziness and difficulty concentrating, that they decided to seek medical advice.

At first, Pat's doctors suspected common conditions like migraines or tension headaches. Neurological tests were ordered, and medications were prescribed, but nothing seemed to help. It wasn't until Pat's mother insisted on further investigation, refusing to accept that nothing was wrong, that the doctors began to consider more serious possibilities. Her story, like many others with Chiari, underscores the importance of advocating for oneself or one's child when the answers aren't clear.

Diagnostic Tests for Chiari Malformation

There are several key tests that are typically involved in diagnosing Chiari Malformation, but it's worth noting that not every path to diagnosis is straightforward. For some, like Pat, a single test can provide the answers, while for others, it takes multiple tests and second opinions.

1. **Magnetic Resonance Imaging (MRI):** The MRI is the gold standard for diagnosing Chiari Malformation. It provides detailed images of the brain and spinal cord, allowing doctors to see the position of the cerebellar tonsils (the part of the brain that herniates into the spinal canal in Chiari). An MRI can reveal the degree of tonsillar herniation, which is crucial in confirming the diagnosis. In Pat's case, after months of inconclusive tests, her neurologist finally ordered an MRI of the brain and cervical spine. The results showed that Pat had Type I Chiari Malformation, with her cerebellar tonsils extending into her spinal canal by several millimeters.

2. **Cine MRI:** A cine MRI is a specialized form of MRI that measures cerebrospinal fluid (CSF) flow around the brain and spinal cord. Chiari Malformation can obstruct the normal flow of CSF, causing pressure on the brain and spinal cord, which leads to many of the symptoms associated with the condition. For Pat, the cine MRI was particularly important because it revealed that her Chiari was not only causing her headaches but also affecting her CSF flow. This discovery played a significant role in her treatment plan.

3.   **CT Scan:** Although less common for diagnosing Chiari, a CT scan can sometimes be used to get a clearer view of bone structures in the skull and spine. It is particularly useful if there is suspicion of associated conditions like basilar invagination (when the top of the spine pushes into the skull), which can occur alongside Chiari.

4.   **Neurological Exam:** While imaging tests are critical, neurological exams are often the first step in the diagnostic process. These exams assess balance, coordination, muscle strength, reflexes, and sensation to determine if the brainstem or spinal cord is being affected. For Pat, these exams helped identify subtle deficits in her coordination and balance, which further supported the need for imaging studies.

5.   **Spinal Tap (Lumbar Puncture):** Although not typically used to diagnose Chiari itself, a spinal tap can help rule out other conditions, such as infections or increased intracranial pressure. In some cases, it can also measure CSF pressure, but this test is not routine for Chiari patients unless there are concerns about other conditions.

Incidental Diagnosis

Interestingly, not all Chiari diagnoses come after years of struggling with symptoms. Some are found incidentally during imaging tests ordered for other reasons. For instance, a person may receive an MRI for chronic neck pain or after a minor head injury and discover they have Chiari Malformation without even suspecting it. These individuals may or may not experience symptoms, and in some cases, the Chiari may never become problematic. This phenomenon is known as an "incidental diagnosis."

For example, one patient, not unlike Pat, had undergone an MRI after a minor car accident that resulted in whiplash. The doctors were primarily looking for any spinal injuries, but instead, they found that the patient had Type I Chiari. It was a shock, as this individual had never experienced symptoms severe enough to suspect a neurological disorder. The question then became, "What next?" Should they monitor the condition, or intervene before symptoms worsened?

Telling Others About Chiari

One of the most challenging aspects of a Chiari diagnosis is explaining it to others, especially when the symptoms can be vague or misunderstood. Chiari Malformation is not well-known, even among some healthcare providers, which can make it difficult for patients to articulate what they are going through.

When Pat was diagnosed, her mother struggled with how to tell family and friends. Some people dismissed Pat's headaches and dizziness as "normal childhood complaints," while others suggested that she was simply trying to avoid schoolwork. This skepticism only made it harder for Pat, who was already feeling isolated and confused by her diagnosis.

For children, like Pat, explaining Chiari to peers can be even more daunting. Pat found it difficult to talk about her condition with her classmates. They couldn't understand why she sometimes needed to sit out of physical activities or why she occasionally had to miss school for doctor's appointments. Her teachers, though sympathetic, didn't always know how to accommodate her needs either.

Many patients with Chiari, especially those with less visible symptoms, struggle with this. They face skepticism from others who cannot see their pain or understand the neurological underpinnings of the condition. This is why support groups and patient advocacy organizations are so important for Chiari patients and their families. These groups offer a sense of community and understanding that is often missing in day-to-day life.

The Emotional Impact of a Diagnosis

Receiving a Chiari diagnosis can be a double-edged sword.

On one hand, it provides relief—finally, there is a name for the symptoms that have been plaguing the patient. On the other hand, it opens up a whole new world of uncertainties and fears.

For Pat's family, the diagnosis was initially overwhelming. Her mother had never heard of Chiari Malformation before and immediately began researching everything she could about the condition. The more she learned, the more questions she had. Would Pat need surgery? How would this affect her quality of life? Could her symptoms worsen over time?

The uncertainty can be paralyzing. Some patients with Chiari live relatively normal lives with minimal symptoms, while others require surgery or ongoing treatment. The unpredictability of the condition can make it difficult to plan for the future.

Pat's mother remembers the moment the doctor explained the potential outcomes. "We might be able to manage it conservatively for now," the doctor had said, "but if her symptoms get worse, surgery may be necessary." Those words hung in the air, and the possibility of invasive treatment weighed heavily on Pat's family.

Conclusion: Navigating the Diagnostic Journey

Chiari Malformation is a condition that can be challenging to diagnose, with each patient's journey to understanding their condition being unique. From the initial symptoms, through a battery of diagnostic tests, to finally receiving a diagnosis, the process can be long, emotionally taxing, and full of uncertainty. But knowing the name of the condition, as overwhelming as it might be, is the first step toward treatment and management.

For Pat, the diagnosis of Chiari Malformation brought clarity, but it also introduced new challenges. Her family had to navigate not only the medical aspects of the condition but also the social and emotional toll it took on her life. As the narrative continues, we will explore how families, like Pat's, manage the day-to-day reality of living with Chiari and the treatment options that are available.

In the next chapter, we will explore the treatment landscape for Chiari Malformation, from conservative management to surgical intervention, and the factors that influence these decisions. For Pat, these choices were life-changing, and her story is a testament to the resilience of those living with this complex condition.

Chiari Malformation (CM) presents with a range of symptoms that often overlap with other neurological conditions, making diagnosis challenging. Symptoms such as headaches, dizziness, neck pain, and balance issues can be attributed to a variety of other disorders, leading to potential misdiagnosis or delayed diagnosis of CM. Understanding the differential diagnoses, or conditions that share similar symptoms with CM, is crucial for healthcare providers to ensure patients receive the correct treatment. In this chapter, we will explore some common differential diagnoses and share patient stories to illustrate the complexities of diagnosing Chiari Malformation.

Common Differential Diagnoses

1. Migraine Headaches

Migraines are one of the most frequent misdiagnoses for Chiari Malformation. Both conditions can cause severe headaches, often at the back of the head, neck pain, and sensitivity to light or sound. However, migraine headaches tend to be episodic, whereas headaches from CM may worsen with activities that increase intracranial pressure, such as coughing, sneezing, or straining.

Patient Story: Sarah's Journey Sarah, a 34-year-old mother of two, had been suffering from debilitating headaches for years. Her neurologist diagnosed her with migraines and prescribed medications to manage her symptoms. However, Sarah noticed that her headaches often worsened when she coughed or bent over, which didn't align with typical migraine patterns. She also began experiencing balance problems and numbness in her hands. After visiting a new neurologist, Sarah underwent an MRI, which revealed that her headaches were not due to migraines but Chiari Malformation. She underwent decompression surgery, and while her headaches didn't completely disappear, they became much more manageable, and her other symptoms improved significantly.

2. Cervical Spondylosis

Cervical spondylosis, a degenerative condition affecting the spine in the neck, is another condition that can mimic the symptoms of Chiari Malformation. Both conditions can cause neck pain, stiffness, and even neurological symptoms like numbness or tingling in the arms or legs. However, cervical spondylosis is typically caused by age-related wear and tear on the spine, while CM is a congenital condition.

Patient Story: John's Experience John, a 50-year-old construction worker, had been dealing with neck pain and occasional numbness in his fingers for years. His doctor attributed his symptoms to cervical spondylosis, given his physically demanding job and age. He was prescribed physical therapy and pain medications, but the treatments provided only temporary relief. As his symptoms progressed to include dizziness and unsteady gait, John sought a second opinion. A neurologist ordered an MRI, which revealed that in addition to mild cervical spondylosis, John had Chiari Malformation. Surgery helped alleviate his dizziness and improve his balance, though his neck pain from the spondylosis persisted.

3. Multiple Sclerosis (MS)

Multiple Sclerosis is a neurological condition that causes the immune system to attack the protective covering of nerves, leading to a wide range of symptoms, including fatigue, vision problems, difficulty walking, and muscle weakness. Some of these symptoms, particularly balance issues and muscle weakness, overlap with those of Chiari Malformation, which can lead to misdiagnosis.

Patient Story: Emily's Diagnosis Dilemma At 28, Emily was in the prime of her life when she started experiencing numbness in her legs, balance problems, and fatigue. Her primary care doctor referred her to a neurologist, who suspected Multiple Sclerosis based on her symptoms and ordered an MRI. The scan didn't show the typical brain lesions associated with MS, but the neurologist believed it was early in the disease progression. Emily began treatment for MS, but her symptoms continued to worsen. She sought a second opinion from another neurologist who took a closer look at her MRI and noted cerebellar tonsil herniation, leading to a diagnosis of Chiari Malformation. Once diagnosed correctly, Emily underwent surgery, which greatly improved her mobility and reduced her symptoms.

4. Syringomyelia

Syringomyelia, a condition where a fluid-filled cyst (syrinx) forms within the spinal cord, often occurs alongside Chiari Malformation but can also exist as a separate condition. Syringomyelia can cause similar symptoms, including chronic pain, muscle weakness, and sensory disturbances. Distinguishing between the two conditions can be difficult, especially because they frequently occur together.

Patient Story: David's Unexpected Discovery David, a 45-year-old athlete, noticed increasing weakness and numbness in his arms, alongside chronic neck pain. His doctor suspected a pinched nerve or a herniated disc and ordered an MRI. The scan revealed a syrinx in his spinal cord, and David was diagnosed with syringomyelia. It wasn't until a neurosurgeon recommended a follow-up MRI that a subtle Chiari Malformation was discovered as the underlying cause of his syringomyelia. Decompression surgery successfully alleviated the pressure on David's brainstem and spinal cord, helping to reduce the size of the syrinx and improve his symptoms.

5. Ehlers-Danlos Syndrome (EDS)

Ehlers-Danlos Syndrome is a connective tissue disorder that affects the skin, joints, and blood vessels, often causing joint hypermobility, skin that bruises easily, and chronic pain. Some individuals with EDS also develop craniocervical instability, which can mimic the symptoms of Chiari Malformation, such as headaches, neck pain, and neurological issues. EDS patients are also at a higher risk of developing Chiari Malformation, making it crucial for healthcare providers to carefully assess symptoms and perform the necessary imaging studies to differentiate between the two conditions.

Patient Story: Rachel's Complex Case Rachel had always been flexible, often showing off her ability to bend her fingers and joints in unusual ways. However, as she grew older, her hypermobility began causing her joint pain and frequent dislocations. She was diagnosed with Ehlers-Danlos Syndrome, and for years she managed her symptoms with physical therapy. When she started experiencing severe headaches and numbness in her limbs, her doctors initially believed these new symptoms were part of her EDS. An MRI later revealed that Rachel also had Chiari Malformation, which was contributing to her worsening neurological symptoms. With the right treatment plan, including surgery for her Chiari Malformation and ongoing management of her EDS, Rachel found significant relief.

6. Idiopathic Intracranial Hypertension (IIH)

Idiopathic Intracranial Hypertension (IIH) is a condition characterized by elevated pressure in the brain without an apparent cause. Like Chiari Malformation, IIH can cause headaches, vision problems, and pulsatile tinnitus (ringing in the ears). The key difference is that IIH typically does not involve herniation of the cerebellar tonsils, and patients with IIH often have normal MRI scans. However, a small percentage of patients with IIH can develop mild cerebellar tonsil herniation, which can complicate diagnosis.

Patient Story: Melissa's Misdiagnosis Melissa, a 25-

year-old recent college graduate, had been struggling with headaches, blurry vision, and a constant ringing in her ears for months. Her ophthalmologist noticed swelling in her optic nerves, a hallmark sign of increased intracranial pressure, and referred her to a neurologist. Based on her symptoms and MRI results showing mild cerebellar tonsil herniation, Melissa was diagnosed with Chiari Malformation. However, her symptoms continued to worsen, and further tests revealed that she actually had Idiopathic Intracranial Hypertension, not CM. Once diagnosed with IIH, Melissa was treated with medication to lower her intracranial pressure, and her symptoms gradually improved.

7. Tethered Cord Syndrome

Tethered Cord Syndrome is a neurological disorder where the spinal cord is abnormally attached to tissues within the spine, limiting its movement. This condition can cause symptoms similar to those of Chiari Malformation, including lower back pain, leg weakness, and sensory disturbances. Tethered Cord Syndrome is often seen in conjunction with Chiari Malformation, but it can also be a standalone condition.

Patient Story: Michael's Confusing Diagnosis Michael, a 13-year-old boy, had been experiencing frequent falls, leg weakness, and pain in his lower back. His pediatrician suspected a musculoskeletal issue and referred him to a neurologist for further evaluation. An MRI revealed both Chiari Malformation and a tethered spinal cord, which was pulling on his spinal nerves and contributing to his symptoms. After undergoing surgery to release his tethered cord, Michael's symptoms improved, though he still requires ongoing monitoring for his Chiari Malformation.

The Importance of Accurate Diagnosis

These patient stories highlight the complexities of diagnosing Chiari Malformation. The overlap in symptoms with other neurological conditions can lead to misdiagnosis or delayed diagnosis, which may prevent patients from receiving the appropriate treatment in a timely manner. For many patients, the journey to a correct diagnosis involves multiple doctor visits, second opinions, and extensive testing.

An accurate diagnosis of Chiari Malformation often requires advanced imaging techniques, such as MRI, and a thorough evaluation by a specialist experienced in CM and related conditions. It is essential to differentiate CM from other neurological disorders to determine the best course of treatment and provide relief from debilitating symptoms.

Diagnostic Tools and Techniques

While MRI remains the gold standard for diagnosing Chiari Malformation, additional tests may be necessary to rule out or confirm other conditions. These may include:

- **CT scans** to evaluate bony structures of the skull and cervical spine.

- **Cine MRI** to assess cerebrospinal fluid (CSF) flow and detect obstructions caused by the cerebellar tonsils.

- **Neurological exams** to assess motor and sensory function, which can help differentiate between conditions like MS and CM.

- **Lumbar puncture** to measure intracranial pressure, particularly in cases where IIH is suspected.

The process of obtaining an accurate diagnosis can be lengthy and frustrating, but it is a crucial step in ensuring that patients receive the correct treatment for their condition.

5 Treatment Options

When faced with a diagnosis of Chiari malformation, one of the most challenging decisions patients and their families face is determining the right course of treatment. Chiari, while potentially debilitating, has varied degrees of severity. Some individuals live their entire lives with minimal symptoms, while others experience significant neurological challenges. This variability in symptoms leads to one of the most debated questions in the treatment of Chiari malformation: should you opt for surgery or take a "wait and see" approach?

Assessing Symptoms: The First Step

The decision to operate is never taken lightly, and it largely depends on the symptoms and their severity. For some, the symptoms of Chiari malformation can be relatively mild, including occasional headaches, neck pain, or dizziness. These symptoms can be manageable with over-the-counter pain relief and lifestyle adjustments. In other cases, symptoms are more severe, affecting balance, motor skills, and cognitive function. These more pronounced symptoms often lead to the need for more aggressive treatment options, including surgery.

However, the decision to move forward with surgery isn't solely based on symptoms. The presence of other associated conditions, such as syringomyelia (a fluid-filled cyst in the spinal cord) or hydrocephalus (an accumulation of cerebrospinal fluid in the brain), may also weigh heavily on the decision to operate. Neurosurgeons take a careful approach, weighing the risks and benefits of surgery, while also considering the patient's age, overall health, and the potential for symptom progression.

For Pat, my friend's daughter, the decision to pursue surgery was a difficult one. At the time of her diagnosis, she was experiencing a combination of severe headaches, dizziness, and difficulty concentrating in school. Her grades, once strong, began to slip, and her energy levels plummeted. As her symptoms worsened, it became clear that waiting was not an option.

The Wait-and-See Approach

For patients with less severe symptoms, the "wait and see" approach is often the first recommendation. This strategy involves regular monitoring by a neurologist or neurosurgeon, keeping track of any changes in symptoms, and undergoing periodic MRIs to ensure there is no worsening of the malformation or the development of associated conditions.

While the idea of "waiting" may sound passive, it is often the best choice when the risks of surgery outweigh the potential benefits. Chiari decompression surgery, while generally safe, carries risks like any major operation. These risks can include infection, nerve damage, and complications related to anesthesia. In cases where symptoms are stable and not significantly impacting daily life, surgery may not be necessary at all.

Pat's mother was initially hopeful that a conservative, wait-and-see approach might be enough. But Pat's symptoms, which had been manageable at first, escalated rapidly. Her mother noticed that she was having trouble with tasks that had never been an issue before—holding a pencil, balancing on one leg during gym class, even walking straight without tripping. The once vibrant and active girl became more withdrawn, quiet, and fatigued.

Their neurosurgeon recommended close monitoring, but after just a few months of escalating symptoms, it became clear that waiting was no longer a safe option. The decision was made to move forward with surgery.

Finding the Right Neurosurgeon

Finding the right neurosurgeon is crucial when deciding on surgery. Chiari malformation is a complex condition, and not all neurosurgeons are equally experienced in its treatment. It's important to seek out a specialist who has a track record of successfully treating Chiari patients, someone who understands the nuances of the condition and its associated complications.

Pat's family was fortunate to find a highly recommended pediatric neurosurgeon with extensive experience in Chiari decompression surgery. The surgeon spent a considerable amount of time explaining the procedure, the risks involved, and the potential outcomes. This transparency allowed Pat's family to make an informed decision, knowing that while surgery could alleviate her symptoms, it was not a guaranteed cure.

The Surgery: What to Expect

Chiari decompression surgery is the most common procedure used to treat Chiari malformation. The goal of the surgery is to relieve pressure on the brain and spinal cord by creating more space for the cerebellum at the base of the skull. This is typically achieved by removing a small portion of the bone at the back of the skull (called a craniectomy) and sometimes removing part of the first cervical vertebra. In some cases, the surgeon may also open the dura, a protective membrane around the brain, and add a patch to further enlarge the space.

For patients like Pat, the surgery is often seen as the best hope for relieving symptoms. However, it is not without risks. The recovery process can be long, and the outcome is not always predictable. Some patients experience significant relief from symptoms almost immediately, while others may have a slower recovery or continue to deal with lingering symptoms.

Pat's surgery took place early in the morning. Her family arrived at the hospital before sunrise, and though they had been preparing for this day for weeks, the reality of the situation hit them all at once. Her mother struggled to keep her composure, while Pat, at just ten years old, was remarkably calm. She didn't fully understand the gravity of the situation, but she knew she would be "fixed" after the surgery—at least, that was how her young mind processed it.

The surgery lasted several hours, during which her parents waited anxiously, praying for good news. When the neurosurgeon finally came out to speak with them, he reassured them that the procedure had gone as expected, but that Pat's recovery would require patience and vigilance.

Post-Surgery Recovery

Recovery from Chiari surgery can vary from person to person. In most cases, patients will spend several days in the hospital, closely monitored for any signs of complications. Pain management is a critical part of the early recovery process, as the surgery itself can cause significant discomfort, especially around the neck and head.

Pat's recovery was challenging, as it is for many children who undergo such an invasive procedure. The first few days after the surgery were spent in the Pediatric Intensive Care Unit (PICU), where she was hooked up to various monitors, an IV drip, and a morphine pump to control her pain. Her mother stayed by her side, comforting her and making sure the nurses were always nearby.

The pain was intense, and Pat often felt nauseous from the anesthesia and pain medications. Her mother described the experience as "gut-wrenching" but knew it was necessary for Pat's long-term health.

Once Pat was moved out of the PICU and into a regular hospital room, her recovery progressed more slowly. She had to relearn how to move her head without experiencing searing pain, and her energy levels were still low. Physical therapy became a crucial part of her rehabilitation, helping her regain her strength and mobility.

Despite the difficulties, there were glimmers of hope. Within a few weeks, Pat's headaches, which had once been so debilitating, began to lessen. The dizziness that had plagued her for months subsided, and her balance began to improve. It wasn't an overnight transformation, but the small victories gave her family hope that the surgery had been the right decision.

When It's Your Child with Chiari

When the person suffering from Chiari malformation is a child, the weight of the decision to operate is even greater. For parents, watching their child endure such pain and uncertainty is nothing short of agonizing. But the decision to pursue surgery is often driven by the understanding that the alternative—allowing symptoms to worsen unchecked—could lead to a significantly reduced quality of life.

Pat's mother often talks about the emotional toll the experience took on her. The days leading up to the surgery were filled with anxiety and doubt, and the recovery process was fraught with moments of second-guessing. But now, years later, she can look back and say with certainty that the surgery gave her daughter a chance at a normal life.

"Seeing your child suffer is the worst thing a parent can go through," Pat's mother said. "But you have to have faith. Faith in the doctors, faith in the process, and faith that you're making the right decision."

Moving Forward with Hope

Today, Pat is thriving. Her recovery took time, but she returned to school, resumed her favorite activities, and regained her strength. She still deals with occasional symptoms, but the most debilitating ones are behind her. For Pat and her family, the decision to move forward with surgery, though difficult, was ultimately the right one.

For families facing the decision to operate on their child's Chiari malformation, the road ahead may seem daunting. But with the right support, a skilled neurosurgeon, and faith in the process, there is hope for a brighter future.

Every case of Chiari malformation is unique, and the decision to operate should always be made in consultation with a qualified medical professional. For some, surgery is a clear path forward. For others, a more conservative approach may be best. But in all cases, the focus should remain on improving the patient's quality of life and managing symptoms in a way that allows them to live as fully as possible.

In the next chapters, we will explore the long-term outlook for individuals with Chiari malformation and how to manage the condition in everyday life. Whether you choose surgery or a more conservative route, understanding the road ahead can make all the difference.

When it comes to Chiari malformation, the question of outcomes is central to understanding both the effectiveness of treatments and the overall prognosis for patients. While Chiari malformation is often described as a structural abnormality of the brain, the range of symptoms and their severity can vary greatly from one person to another. Because of this variability, measuring outcomes after diagnosis, treatment, and especially surgery can be complex.

In this chapter, we will explore how outcomes are measured, the different paths patients take depending on their treatment decisions, and what happens when surgery doesn't yield the expected results. We'll also revisit Pat's story to understand how her journey has been shaped by the outcomes of the decisions made at different stages.

How Outcomes Are Measured

The primary goal of Chiari malformation treatment is symptom relief, but the path to achieving this varies. Before diving into the specifics of surgical outcomes, it's important to understand how doctors and patients measure success.

Outcomes are often classified into several categories:

- **Symptom Relief**: The reduction or complete disappearance of symptoms such as headaches, neck pain, balance issues, and more severe neurological problems.

- **Neurological Function**: Restoring or maintaining proper neurological function is one of the most critical markers of a positive outcome. This includes regaining lost motor skills or improving coordination and balance.

- **Quality of Life**: For many patients, quality of life is a critical measure of success. How well they can return to normal activities—working, exercising, socializing—is as important as any clinical metric.

- **Long-term Stability**: Even if short-term symptoms are improved, long-term stability is crucial. Doctors want to ensure that the Chiari malformation doesn't worsen over time or cause new issues such as syringomyelia, a buildup of fluid in the spinal cord.

- **MRI Findings**: Imaging tests such as MRIs are essential in assessing the anatomical changes after surgery or treatment. A positive outcome might be shown by improved cerebrospinal fluid (CSF) flow or reduction in herniation.

Each of these outcomes is vital in evaluating the effectiveness of treatment, but patients and their families may prioritize them differently depending on their unique situations.

Wait-and-See Outcomes

Not every Chiari malformation diagnosis leads immediately to surgery. In many cases, doctors recommend a conservative approach known as "wait and see," particularly for patients with mild or manageable symptoms. This involves careful monitoring through regular MRIs and neurological exams to track whether the condition progresses.

For some patients, this approach works well. Symptoms may remain stable for years or may worsen so gradually that surgery is never necessary. A "wait-and-see" outcome is generally considered successful if the patient's symptoms remain manageable without intervention.

However, this approach also carries risks. Symptoms can worsen unexpectedly, or complications such as syringomyelia can develop without warning. If this happens, doctors may need to intervene with surgery, sometimes under more urgent circumstances than if surgery had been performed earlier.

Pat's Experience with the Wait-and-See Approach

Pat's family initially decided to take the "wait-and-see" approach after her diagnosis. At that point, her symptoms were minimal—mostly mild headaches and occasional dizziness. Her doctors believed that her young age might allow her to manage the symptoms without surgery, and for a time, this seemed like a good decision.

For about a year after her diagnosis, Pat's condition remained stable. She went to school, played with friends, and led a relatively normal life. Her mother, however, was always watching for signs of progression. Every headache, every moment of dizziness sent her into a spiral of worry.

Despite the relatively stable condition during this period, Pat's symptoms eventually began to worsen. What were once mild headaches turned into severe migraines that would leave her bedridden for days. Her balance problems also grew more noticeable, and she started to miss school due to her inability to concentrate. At this point, the decision to move forward with surgery became inevitable.

Surgical Outcomes

For many patients, surgery is the most definitive treatment for Chiari malformation. The most common surgery, known as posterior fossa decompression, involves removing a small portion of bone at the back of the skull to relieve pressure and restore the normal flow of CSF.

The outcomes of surgery can be life-changing for many patients, with a significant percentage experiencing immediate relief from debilitating symptoms. However, the results are not always so clear-cut, and there are several factors that can affect surgical outcomes:

- **Timing of Surgery**: Early surgical intervention often leads to better outcomes, particularly if symptoms are severe. The longer nerve damage persists, the less likely it is that neurological function can be fully restored.

- **Age and Overall Health**: Younger patients, like Pat, tend to have better surgical outcomes compared to older patients. Additionally, overall health plays a role in how well a patient recovers.

- **Complications During Surgery**: As with any surgery, there are risks. Complications such as infections, cerebrospinal fluid leaks, or improper healing can affect outcomes.

- **Extent of Decompression**: Some patients may require more extensive surgery to relieve pressure, particularly if there are additional complications such as syringomyelia or tethered cord syndrome.

For many, surgery can offer substantial relief. In some cases, headaches disappear entirely, balance issues improve, and neurological function is restored. Many patients find that their quality of life dramatically improves after surgery.

However, it's important to understand that surgery is not a guaranteed cure. While it may improve symptoms, the malformation itself remains, and the goal is to manage its impact rather than eliminate it entirely.

Pat's Surgical Experience

Pat's surgery was a difficult decision for her family. After months of watching her struggle with worsening symptoms, her parents were finally ready to move forward with the procedure. Pat, too, had grown tired of the constant headaches and the limitations they placed on her daily life.

The day of surgery was fraught with anxiety for everyone. While her neurosurgeon was confident, Pat's mother couldn't help but worry about the risks. What if something went wrong? What if surgery didn't help? These were questions that swirled in her mind as they waited in the hospital's sterile, impersonal waiting room.

Thankfully, the surgery went smoothly. Pat's recovery was difficult at first, with weeks of pain and discomfort. However, as the swelling subsided and her body began to heal, it became clear that the surgery had been a success. Pat's headaches became less frequent, her balance improved, and she returned to school with a newfound sense of normalcy.

For Pat and her family, surgery was the turning point they had hoped for. It wasn't a perfect fix—she still had to be cautious and manage her health carefully—but it gave her back much of the life she had been missing.

When Surgery Fails

While many patients experience positive outcomes after surgery, there are cases where surgery does not bring the relief that was expected. In some instances, patients may continue to experience symptoms, or new ones may emerge. This can happen for several reasons:

- **Incomplete Decompression**: If the decompression does not adequately relieve pressure or restore CSF flow, symptoms may persist or worsen.

- **Scar Tissue Formation**: Scar tissue can develop after surgery, leading to renewed pressure on the brainstem or spinal cord.

- **Syringomyelia**: Even after decompression surgery, some patients develop syringomyelia, which can cause ongoing pain, weakness, and neurological issues.

- **Misdiagnosis or Multiple Conditions**: In some cases, the underlying cause of the symptoms may not be fully addressed by the surgery, especially if the patient has multiple overlapping conditions, such as tethered cord syndrome or Ehlers-Danlos syndrome.

When surgery fails, patients may need additional interventions. Some may undergo a second decompression surgery, while others turn to alternative therapies or pain management techniques. It can be a frustrating and disheartening experience, but it's important for patients and their families to understand that setbacks are part of the journey for some.

Pat's Journey Forward

Pat's surgery was a success, but she knew other children who weren't as fortunate. She met some of them through online support groups, and their stories were a stark reminder that not everyone experiences a smooth recovery. For Pat, it was important to acknowledge her good fortune, but she also felt a deep empathy for those still struggling.

Her mother, too, found solace in these online communities. Connecting with other parents who had faced the same difficult decisions provided a support network that had been missing when they first started this journey.

Pat's story, while one of relative success, is a testament to the varied outcomes that can come from Chiari malformation. Her journey was not without its struggles, and the decision to undergo surgery was one of the hardest her family had to make. But in the end, it gave her the relief she desperately needed.

Conclusion

Outcomes in Chiari malformation are diverse and can depend on numerous factors, including the timing of intervention, the type of surgery performed, and the presence of complicating conditions. For many, surgery offers relief and a return to normalcy, but for others, it can be the beginning of a long and challenging road.

Recovery from Chiari malformation surgery is a significant and often challenging process. It requires patience, resilience, and, most importantly, support from loved ones and medical professionals. While the outcome of surgery may alleviate many symptoms, recovery is not immediate, and it's important to understand what to expect, both physically and emotionally, during this critical phase. For some, recovery can be smooth with minor setbacks, while others may face a longer, more difficult journey.

In this chapter, we'll explore the general recovery process after Chiari surgery, what symptoms to expect during this period, and how to make the most of a support system. Additionally, we'll dive into Pat's personal recovery story—her physical and emotional journey following surgery—to provide an insightful look into what recovery can entail for a child and her family.

The Recovery Process: An Overview

Recovering from Chiari surgery is often a lengthy process that can take several months or even longer. The road to recovery depends on multiple factors, including the individual's overall health, the severity of symptoms before surgery, and the specific type of surgery performed.

Immediate Post-Surgery Recovery

Immediately following Chiari decompression surgery, patients are typically monitored in a recovery room or intensive care unit (ICU). This monitoring is critical to ensure that there are no complications from the surgery, such as excessive bleeding or infection. Patients may experience some disorientation from anesthesia and discomfort at the surgical site, especially around the neck and head.

Pain management is an important part of the early recovery phase. Doctors often prescribe medications to control the pain, including opioids or non-steroidal anti-inflammatory drugs (NSAIDs). Ice packs may also be applied to the surgical area to reduce swelling and discomfort.

Some patients may have a drain inserted at the surgical site to help reduce excess fluid buildup, which is removed within a day or two. Nurses and medical staff carefully monitor the patient for signs of cerebrospinal fluid (CSF) leakage or any infection.

First Week Post-Surgery

For most people, the first week after Chiari surgery is the most physically demanding. Neck stiffness and headaches are common during this period, along with some difficulty in moving the head. Physical therapy may be introduced early on to encourage gentle movements, helping to prevent long-term stiffness. It's crucial to follow medical advice on how much movement is safe during the early stages of recovery, as overexertion can lead to complications or delays in healing.

Patients are usually discharged within a week, but only after demonstrating stable vitals and an ability to manage pain at home. In Pat's case, after her surgery, she had to stay in the hospital for several days longer than expected due to mild swelling near her incision site. Her mother, who had been with her every day, described those initial days as a "roller coaster of emotions." Watching Pat struggle with pain and fatigue after surgery was heart-wrenching, but it was also a reminder of how much progress she had made in addressing the severe symptoms that once ruled her life.

Physical Symptoms During Recovery

It's common for patients to experience some of the following symptoms in the weeks after surgery:

Headaches

Headaches are one of the most frequent symptoms patients experience during recovery. While decompression surgery aims to relieve pressure on the brainstem and spinal cord, it can take weeks or even months for the body to fully adjust to these changes. Headaches may persist, especially in the early stages of recovery. Pain medications can help alleviate the intensity, and patients are often advised to rest in a quiet, low-stress environment to minimize any triggers.

Neck Pain and Stiffness

Due to the surgical procedure, neck pain and stiffness are common side effects. The muscles and tissues around the incision site need time to heal, and this often results in limited mobility for several weeks. Physical therapy plays a key role in helping to regain strength and flexibility, but exercises should be performed cautiously to avoid overextending the neck.

Pat experienced significant neck pain after her surgery, particularly during the first two weeks at home. Her parents helped her with gentle neck exercises and provided extra pillows to support her head while she rested. Though the pain was difficult, Pat's mother noted that the worst of it passed after the first month, and they saw a gradual improvement in her ability to move comfortably.

Fatigue

Fatigue is another common symptom post-surgery. It's important to remember that the body is working hard to heal, and this requires energy. Many patients find they are easily tired in the weeks following surgery and may need to sleep more than usual. Simple tasks like walking around the house or sitting up for extended periods can feel exhausting.

In Pat's case, fatigue was particularly challenging. Her

energy levels were low for the first few weeks, and she often needed extra naps during the day. Her mother explained that it was important not to rush Pat's recovery and to allow her plenty of time to rest and regain her strength.

Sensory Issues

Some patients experience sensory disturbances during recovery, such as numbness, tingling, or weakness in the arms and legs. These symptoms may stem from the changes in pressure around the brainstem and spinal cord. While they often resolve over time, some individuals may need physical therapy to help restore normal function.

The Emotional Side of Recovery

Recovering from Chiari surgery isn't just about physical healing—it's also about emotional recovery. The surgery itself can be a frightening and overwhelming experience, and the recovery period may bring about feelings of frustration, fear, or even depression. It's not uncommon for patients to feel isolated, especially if their mobility is limited or if they are unable to return to their normal routine.

Emotional Support for Children and Families

For children like Pat, the recovery process is particularly difficult. Pat's surgery took place when she was young, and while she was a brave little girl, there were days when her emotions ran high. Her mother recalled the moments when Pat would cry out of frustration, unable to understand why recovery wasn't faster or easier. "She'd ask, 'Why does it still hurt, Mom?' and it broke my heart every time," her mother said.

Supporting a child through recovery means addressing not just the physical symptoms but also the emotional toll. Pat's parents focused on creating a calm, comforting environment where Pat felt safe. They filled her days with activities that didn't require too much energy—reading books, doing simple crafts, and watching her favorite movies. It also helped that her parents reassured her that it was okay to feel upset or tired.

For parents, watching their child recover can feel overwhelming. It's important to seek support from other parents or professionals who understand the challenges of post-surgery recovery. Talking to a counselor or joining a support group can provide much-needed encouragement and guidance.

Using Your Support System

Recovery from Chiari surgery is not a solo endeavor. It requires a strong support system made up of family, friends, medical professionals, and, when necessary, specialized support groups.

Lean on Family and Friends

One of the most critical elements of recovery is the help and encouragement from loved ones. Whether it's assisting with daily tasks, managing medications, or simply offering emotional support, family and friends play a crucial role in recovery. For those recovering from surgery, asking for help can be difficult, but it's essential for maintaining progress. When Pat was recovering, her grandparents came to visit and helped with meals and cleaning around the house, allowing her parents to focus on her needs.

Communicate with Healthcare Providers

Consistent communication with healthcare providers is key to ensuring a successful recovery. Doctors, physical therapists, and nurses can provide valuable guidance on managing symptoms, monitoring progress, and avoiding potential complications. Regular follow-up appointments are also crucial for tracking recovery milestones and addressing any concerns that arise.

Online and In-Person Support Groups

Many patients and families find that connecting with others who have experienced Chiari malformation and its treatments is incredibly helpful. Whether through online forums, local support groups, or national organizations, these communities provide a safe space to share stories, ask questions, and offer support. Pat's mother joined a Chiari support group online, where she found comfort in hearing from other parents who had gone through similar experiences with their children.

Pat's Recovery Journey

Pat's journey of recovery was not without its challenges. After being discharged from the hospital, she faced weeks of limited mobility and frequent discomfort. For the first month, her parents had to help her with daily activities like dressing, brushing her hair, and walking short distances. She was unable to return to school for several weeks, which left her feeling disconnected from her friends and classmates.

But over time, Pat made gradual improvements. Her headaches became less frequent, her neck pain eased, and she slowly regained her strength. By the third month post-surgery, Pat was able to attend school part-time and even joined her friends for light activities at recess. Her family celebrated each small victory, knowing that recovery is a process that takes time.

Pat's mother emphasized that having faith and patience was key to her daughter's recovery. "It wasn't easy, but we just took it one day at a time. We kept reminding Pat—and ourselves—that healing is slow, but it's worth it."

Looking Ahead

The recovery process after Chiari surgery is unique for every individual, but the key themes remain the same: patience, support, and the recognition that healing takes time. With the right approach, many people, like Pat, are able to regain a sense of normalcy and lead fulfilling lives after surgery. In the next chapter, we will explore what it's like to live with Chiari after surgery, the potential long-term effects, and how patients can continue to manage their condition in the years to come.

Living with Chiari malformation is not simply a medical diagnosis; it's a way of life that impacts nearly every aspect of an individual's existence. For those affected, every day brings its own unique set of challenges—from the physical pain that can be relentless, to the emotional toll it takes on families and relationships, to the impact it has on school, work, and even pregnancy. In this chapter, we'll explore what it means to live with Chiari malformation, with a focus on how it affects everyday life, and share how several patients navigated the complexities of living with this condition.

The Physical Impact of Pain

Pain is one of the most significant challenges faced by people living with Chiari malformation. Headaches, neck pain, dizziness, and muscle weakness are common symptoms that can flare up at any time, making it difficult to engage in normal activities. For some, the pain may be intermittent and manageable, but for others, it can be a constant companion that limits their ability to function. In either case, it's critical for those with Chiari to learn how to manage their pain effectively.

Pat's experience is a testament to the importance of pain management. As a child, she was active and full of energy, but as her Chiari symptoms worsened, she began to experience debilitating headaches that left her bedridden for days. Her parents quickly realized that pain management wasn't just about medication—it was about understanding her limits. Pat's doctors developed a pain management plan that combined medication with physical therapy, and over time, she learned to listen to her body, pacing herself and recognizing when she needed to rest.

For many living with Chiari, the key to managing pain is finding a balance between activity and rest. Staying active is important for maintaining physical strength and overall health, but overexertion can lead to symptom flare-ups. A tailored exercise program, developed in consultation with a healthcare provider, can help individuals with Chiari stay active without aggravating their symptoms.

In addition to physical therapy and exercise, other non-medical approaches like mindfulness meditation, deep breathing exercises, and biofeedback have proven beneficial for some individuals. These techniques can help reduce stress, which is known to exacerbate pain and other Chiari symptoms.

The Family Impact: Supporting a Loved One with Chiari

When someone is diagnosed with Chiari, the impact on their family can be profound. Chiari malformation is a complex and often misunderstood condition, and watching a loved one suffer through pain and uncertainty can be difficult. Family members often take on the role of caregiver, managing doctor appointments, medications, and treatments, while also providing emotional support.

For Pat's family, her diagnosis marked the beginning of a long journey that affected everyone in the household. Her parents were initially overwhelmed by the medical jargon and the uncertain prognosis, but they quickly became her strongest advocates. They learned everything they could about the condition, sought out specialists, and created a support network of friends, teachers, and healthcare providers who could help Pat succeed. Pat's siblings also had to adjust to the new reality. At times, they felt left out when their parents' attention was focused on Pat's health, but over time, they learned that supporting her was a family effort.

Family dynamics often shift when one member has a chronic condition, and open communication is essential. Siblings may feel jealous of the attention given to the affected child, while parents may feel guilty for not being able to do more. It's important for families to talk openly about these feelings and work together to find solutions that support everyone's emotional health.

Support groups, both online and in person, can be invaluable for families living with Chiari. These groups provide a space to share experiences, seek advice, and connect with others who understand the challenges. Many families find comfort in knowing they are not alone in their journey.

Chiari and Education: Navigating School with a Chronic Condition

For children and teens with Chiari, school can present a unique set of challenges. The physical symptoms, particularly chronic pain and fatigue, can make it difficult to concentrate, complete homework, and participate in extracurricular activities. Frequent doctor's appointments and the need for rest may also lead to missed school days, which can affect academic performance.

Pat faced many of these challenges. As her symptoms worsened, she struggled to keep up with her classmates, especially during flare-ups when her headaches were particularly severe. Fortunately, her school was supportive, and with the help of an individualized education plan (IEP), Pat was able to get the accommodations she needed to succeed. She was given extra time for assignments, allowed to rest in a quiet room during the day when she felt overwhelmed, and provided with notes from teachers when she had to miss class.

For children like Pat, early intervention and collaboration between parents, teachers, and healthcare providers are critical. IEPs or 504 Plans can be tailored to meet the specific needs of a child with Chiari, providing accommodations such as modified workloads, additional breaks, or flexible scheduling. School counselors and nurses can also play a key role in ensuring that students with Chiari have the support they need to thrive academically and emotionally.

Parents should advocate for their children's rights in the education system and be open about their child's condition with school staff. It can also be helpful to educate teachers and peers about Chiari malformation, as understanding the condition can foster a more supportive and compassionate environment.

The Impact on Work: Managing Chiari in the Workplace

For adults with Chiari, managing the condition in the workplace can be a significant challenge. The unpredictability of symptoms, particularly headaches and dizziness, can make it difficult to maintain a consistent work schedule. Some individuals may need to reduce their hours or switch to a more flexible job, while others may require accommodations to help manage their symptoms.

Pat's mother, who worked full-time as a teacher, found herself struggling to balance her career and caring for her daughter. She requested a more flexible schedule so that she could be available for doctor's appointments and to help Pat manage her symptoms at home. For Pat's mother, being open with her employer about the challenges of having a child with Chiari allowed her to maintain her job while also being there for her daughter.

In the workplace, individuals with Chiari may qualify for accommodations under the Americans with Disabilities Act (ADA). Accommodations could include flexible work hours, the ability to work from home during flare-ups, ergonomic adjustments to reduce pain, or time off for medical appointments. It's important for individuals with Chiari to have an open conversation with their employer about their needs and to understand their rights under the ADA.

For those who are unable to work due to the severity of

their symptoms, Social Security Disability Insurance (SSDI) may be an option. Applying for disability benefits can be a lengthy process, but with the support of a healthcare provider, many individuals with Chiari are able to successfully secure the financial assistance they need.

Chiari and Pregnancy: What to Expect

Pregnancy can be a time of great joy, but for women with Chiari malformation, it can also be a time of concern. Chiari can complicate pregnancy, particularly for women who have undergone surgery. The increased pressure in the body during pregnancy can exacerbate symptoms, particularly headaches and neck pain. In some cases, the added strain on the body may lead to an increase in neurological symptoms, such as balance issues or dizziness.

Pat's mother recalls the fears she had about whether Pat would be able to have children someday. As she grew older, Pat also wondered what pregnancy would look like for her. While every woman's experience with Chiari and pregnancy is different, it's important for women to work closely with both their neurosurgeon and obstetrician to monitor their symptoms throughout pregnancy. Some women with Chiari may require additional imaging to assess any changes in their condition, while others may need to adjust their medication regimen to ensure the safety of both mother and baby.

For women who have had Chiari decompression surgery, the scar tissue and changes in cerebrospinal fluid (CSF) flow can make delivery more complex. In some cases, a cesarean section may be recommended to reduce the strain on the body during childbirth.

However, with proper monitoring and care, many women with Chiari malformation go on to have healthy pregnancies and children. It's important for women to advocate for themselves, seek the guidance of healthcare providers who are knowledgeable about Chiari, and take steps to manage their symptoms throughout the pregnancy journey.

Patient Stories

Amanda's Journey: Coping with Delayed Diagnosis

Amanda was 28 years old when she started experiencing strange symptoms: headaches, neck pain, and an overwhelming sense of fatigue. She had always been an active person, regularly running and participating in yoga classes. But over time, her energy dwindled, and her once mild headaches turned into severe, throbbing pain that worsened when she coughed or sneezed. Doctors initially brushed off her concerns, attributing her symptoms to stress or tension headaches. For years, she struggled to find relief, feeling frustrated and alone in her search for answers.

It wasn't until Amanda was 32 that she received an MRI and was diagnosed with Chiari Malformation Type I. Learning that her brain had been pushing against her spinal cord for years was both shocking and a relief—it explained everything. Amanda finally had a name for the condition that had been wreaking havoc on her life. But she soon learned that her journey was far from over.

Amanda was recommended for surgery, and although the recovery process was difficult, she eventually found relief from her debilitating headaches. However, her journey with Chiari didn't end there. She continues to experience fatigue and occasional neck pain, and she has had to adjust her expectations for her physical activity levels. Through it all, Amanda found strength in her family and the Chiari community. She now speaks openly about her experience to help others who might be struggling with delayed diagnosis or misdiagnosis. "It took me years to get the right answer," she says, "but I learned to keep advocating for myself. That's what made all the difference."

Javier's Story: From Athlete to Advocate

Javier was a star soccer player throughout high school, dreaming of pursuing a college athletic career. But at age 19, he began to experience symptoms that threatened his future. His once occasional headaches became intense and debilitating. Along with these headaches, Javier noticed that his balance was off, which affected his performance on the field. His coordination seemed to slip, and even everyday tasks felt more challenging. He shrugged it off at first, attributing the symptoms to the strain of playing sports at a competitive level. It wasn't until a particularly bad fall during a game that left him with neck pain that Javier decided to seek medical advice.

After a series of tests, including an MRI, Javier received his diagnosis: Chiari Malformation Type I. The news left him devastated. He had never heard of Chiari before and felt like his world was crashing down. How could he continue to pursue his soccer dreams with a condition that affected his balance, coordination, and caused chronic headaches?

Javier's doctors suggested surgery, but he was hesitant. He worried about how the surgery might impact his ability to play soccer. Ultimately, he decided to go through with the decompression surgery, hoping it would give him a chance to continue doing what he loved. After months of recovery and physical therapy, Javier slowly regained his strength and coordination. While he was able to return to soccer, he knew he wouldn't be able to compete at the same level. His focus shifted, and he channeled his energy into advocating for others with Chiari Malformation.

Today, Javier works as a motivational speaker, sharing his story with young athletes and encouraging them to prioritize their health. "Chiari changed my life," he says, "but it didn't take away my love for the game. It just gave me a new way to play—by helping others find strength and resilience in their challenge."

Lila's Story: A Family's Struggle for Answers

Lila was only eight years old when her parents noticed something was wrong. She was a happy, energetic child, but over time, she began to complain about constant headaches and neck pain. Her parents initially thought it was due to poor posture or too much screen time, but the pain persisted. Soon, Lila started having trouble at school. She became more forgetful and had difficulty concentrating in class. Her grades began to slip, and teachers raised concerns about her ability to stay focused.

Concerned, Lila's parents took her to multiple doctors. They were told she might have migraines or even anxiety, and various medications were prescribed. However, nothing seemed to help. The family felt stuck—unable to understand why their daughter was suffering so much. It wasn't until they saw a neurologist who ordered an MRI that they finally received the diagnosis of Chiari Malformation.

The news was overwhelming for Lila's parents. They were relieved to have an answer, but also scared about what this would mean for their daughter's future. Lila underwent surgery to relieve the pressure on her brain and spinal cord. The recovery process was long, but after several months, her symptoms began to improve. Her headaches became less frequent, and she was able to focus better in school.

Today, Lila is a thriving teenager, though she still experiences occasional symptoms. Her family has become vocal advocates for Chiari awareness, particularly when it comes to educating parents and teachers about the condition. "We want other families to know that they're not alone," Lila's mother says. "It can be a long road to diagnosis, but don't stop searching for answers. Your child's health depends on it."

Martin's Journey: Facing Surgery as an Adult

At 45 years old, Martin had lived with symptoms of Chiari Malformation for decades without knowing it. He had always experienced neck stiffness and occasional headaches but thought they were just part of getting older or from his work as a construction manager. Over time, though, his symptoms worsened. He began to experience a constant pressure in his head, particularly when he strained or bent over. At its worst, the pain was so intense that it left him bedridden.

Martin's symptoms grew more concerning when he started to notice numbness and tingling in his hands and feet. His balance became unpredictable, and he had to stop working due to the risk of falling on the job site. His wife urged him to see a specialist, and after numerous appointments with different doctors, he was finally diagnosed with Chiari Malformation Type I.

The decision to undergo surgery as an adult was a difficult one for Martin. He worried about the risks and whether the surgery would help alleviate his symptoms. However, his quality of life had deteriorated so much that he decided to move forward with decompression surgery. The recovery was long and challenging, but Martin eventually regained much of his previous strength and mobility.

While he still experiences occasional symptoms, such as stiffness in his neck, Martin feels that the surgery was a turning point in his life. He's now more aware of the importance of self-care and pacing himself. "I spent years ignoring my body's warning signs," he says. "I wish I had known about Chiari earlier, but I'm grateful I finally got the help I needed."

Sarah's Struggle: Post-Surgery Challenges

Sarah's journey with Chiari Malformation began in her mid-20s. She had always been prone to headaches, but they intensified as she got older. Eventually, they were accompanied by dizziness, vertigo, and numbness in her extremities. After several visits to her primary care physician and a neurologist, an MRI revealed that Sarah had Chiari Malformation Type I.

Her doctors recommended surgery, and Sarah agreed, hoping it would resolve her symptoms. The surgery went smoothly, and Sarah initially felt some relief. However, within a few months, some of her symptoms returned. The headaches and dizziness came back, though not as severely as before. She was frustrated, having believed that the surgery would be a cure.

Sarah's doctors explained that while decompression surgery is often effective, it doesn't always eliminate all symptoms. In her case, it was possible that her symptoms were related to lingering issues with cerebrospinal fluid flow or nerve damage. After several follow-up appointments and additional testing, Sarah was diagnosed with a condition known as "Chiari Malformation recurrence." She faced the possibility of needing another surgery in the future.

Despite these setbacks, Sarah has learned to manage her symptoms through lifestyle changes, including regular physical therapy, meditation, and a careful approach to physical activity. "I've had to come to terms with the fact that Chiari isn't something that goes away," she says. "But that doesn't mean I'm powerless. I'm learning to live with it and finding ways to take care of myself, even on the hard days."

Ethan's Story: Overcoming Social Isolation

Ethan was 15 when he was diagnosed with Chiari Malformation. He had always been a shy, introverted kid, but after his diagnosis, his social life became even more limited. As his symptoms—headaches, neck pain, and fatigue—intensified, Ethan found it harder to keep up with his friends. He had to stop playing sports, which had once been his favorite activity. He also missed a significant amount of school, and when he was there, he struggled to concentrate in class. His teachers didn't always understand his condition, and neither did his peers. Ethan often felt isolated and misunderstood.

His parents were supportive, but they didn't know how to help him stay connected to his friends and maintain some sense of normalcy. They encouraged him to join an online support group for teens with chronic illness, and it was there that Ethan found a sense of community. For the first time, he was able to connect with other young people who understood what he was going through. He began sharing his story and offering support to others, which helped him feel less alone.

Through his connections in the support group, Ethan also found a new hobby—gaming. He started playing video games with friends online, which became a way for him to stay social, even on days when his symptoms kept him at home. While Chiari Malformation is still a challenge for Ethan, he has found ways to adapt and cope with the social aspects of living with a chronic condition. "It's not easy, but I've learned that there are people out there who understand," he says. "You just have to find your community."

These personal stories illustrate the varied experiences of individuals living with Chiari Malformation, highlighting the unique challenges they face and the resilience they've developed in coping with this complex condition. Whether dealing with delayed diagnoses, navigating surgical outcomes, or managing long-term symptoms, each patient's journey reflects the importance of community, support, and self-advocacy in living with Chiari Malformation.

Conclusion: The Journey Forward

Living with Chiari malformation is a lifelong journey filled with ups and downs. From managing pain to navigating school, work, and family life, those affected by Chiari must learn to balance their symptoms with the demands of everyday life. But with the right support system, medical care, and self-advocacy, it is possible to live a fulfilling life despite the challenges.

For Pat, living with Chiari meant learning to listen to her body, pace herself, and never be afraid to ask for help. She found strength in her family, her healthcare team, and her own resilience, and while Chiari continues to be a part of her life, it does not define her. The next chapter will explore what it means to live with Chiari day-to-day, offering practical tips and guidance for navigating the challenges that lie ahead.

9 Workplace and Educational Challenges

Chiari Malformation (CM) can present a wide range of symptoms, including chronic headaches, dizziness, balance issues, fatigue, and cognitive difficulties. These symptoms can significantly impact various aspects of life, including a person's ability to work and pursue educational opportunities. Both children and adults with CM often face unique challenges in their academic and professional environments, requiring thoughtful adjustments and accommodations. This chapter will explore the workplace and educational challenges faced by individuals with CM and provide strategies to help manage these difficulties while advocating for necessary support.

Understanding the Impact of Chiari Malformation on Work and Education

Chiari Malformation affects individuals in different ways. Some people may experience only mild symptoms and can continue working or attending school with little disruption, while others may be severely affected and require significant adjustments. The nature of the challenges largely depends on the severity of symptoms, the type of work or study being undertaken, and the individual's ability to manage their condition.

Common symptoms of CM that can affect work and school performance include:

- **Chronic headaches**: Frequent or severe headaches can make it difficult to concentrate or complete tasks.

- **Cognitive difficulties**: Memory problems, difficulty concentrating, and slower processing speeds can interfere with learning, problem-solving, and meeting deadlines.

- **Fatigue**: Persistent tiredness can reduce productivity and the ability to engage fully in work or academic tasks.

- **Dizziness and balance issues**: Difficulty with balance can make it challenging to navigate the workplace or school environment safely.

- **Neck pain and stiffness**: Physical discomfort can make it difficult to sit or stand for long periods, impacting job performance or participation in school activities.

- **Visual disturbances**: Blurred vision or double vision can affect reading, working on a computer, and other tasks requiring visual focus.

Given these challenges, it's essential for individuals with CM to develop coping strategies and seek accommodations when necessary to ensure their success in both the workplace and educational settings.

Challenges in the Workplace

People with CM often face specific challenges in the workplace, particularly when their symptoms are unpredictable or worsen over time. The following sections address common issues encountered by employees with CM and offer strategies for managing these challenges.

1. Difficulty Maintaining Consistent Productivity

Frequent headaches, fatigue, and cognitive issues can reduce productivity and make it difficult to meet deadlines or maintain the expected pace of work. Some days may be better than others, leading to variability in performance.

Strategies for Managing Productivity Issues:

- **Pacing and prioritizing**: Break tasks into smaller, manageable chunks and prioritize them based on importance. Allow for breaks to manage symptoms like headaches or fatigue.

- **Flexible scheduling**: If possible, discuss flexible work hours or remote work options with your employer. Being able to work from home on bad days or having the option to adjust work hours can help manage symptoms while still maintaining productivity.

- **Energy conservation**: Use energy-saving techniques, such as delegating tasks when possible or using assistive technology, to reduce the strain of physical and mental work.

2. Physical Discomfort and Environmental Sensitivity

Sitting at a desk for long periods, standing for extended durations, or working in environments with bright lights or loud noises can exacerbate symptoms. Individuals with CM often struggle with neck pain, sensitivity to light, and physical discomfort.

Strategies for Managing Physical Discomfort:

- **Ergonomic adjustments**: Ensure your workspace is ergonomically designed to reduce strain on your neck and back. Adjust your chair, desk height, and computer screen to support good posture.

- **Lighting adjustments**: Request softer lighting or use anti-glare screens to reduce sensitivity to bright lights. Taking breaks from screen work can also alleviate eye strain.

- **Frequent breaks**: Incorporate short breaks into your workday to stretch, move around, and relieve any tension in your neck and back.

- **Assistive devices**: Consider using supportive devices such as a neck brace or lumbar support to manage discomfort while sitting.

3. Absenteeism and Managing Sick Days

Flare-ups of symptoms can lead to increased absenteeism, which can be challenging for both employees and employers. Repeated sick days may cause anxiety about job security or result in missed opportunities for career advancement.

Strategies for Managing Absenteeism:

- **Open communication**: Be transparent with your employer about your condition and how it may impact your attendance. Discuss the possibility of flexible work arrangements or reduced hours if necessary.

- **Use of paid leave**: Familiarize yourself with your company's sick leave policies, including any short-term or long-term disability benefits that may be available to you.

- **Documenting medical needs**: Keep records of medical appointments, doctor's notes, and treatment plans to support any requests for accommodations or time off due to your condition.

4. Stigma and Workplace Perception

Because CM is an invisible illness, colleagues and supervisors may not understand the severity of the condition or how it affects day-to-day functioning. This can lead to misunderstandings or even discrimination in the workplace.

Strategies for Managing Workplace Perception:

- **Advocacy and education**: Educate your employer and co-workers about CM and how it impacts your work. Being open about your challenges can foster understanding and reduce stigma.

- **Know your rights**: Be aware of your legal rights as an employee under the Americans with Disabilities Act (ADA). The ADA requires employers to provide reasonable accommodations for employees with disabilities, including those with chronic illnesses like CM.

Educational Challenges for Students with CM

For children, teens, and adults pursuing education, CM can interfere with their ability to perform academically and participate in school activities. Whether attending elementary school, high school, or university, students with CM may need accommodations to support their learning and ensure they have equal access to educational opportunities.

1. Cognitive Challenges and Learning Difficulties

Cognitive symptoms such as memory problems, difficulty concentrating, and slower information processing can make it challenging to keep up with coursework, complete assignments, and perform well on exams.

Strategies for Managing Cognitive Challenges:

- **Extended time on tests**: Students with CM may qualify for extended time on exams to accommodate slower processing speeds and allow breaks if needed.

- **Note-taking support**: Request assistance with note-taking in class, such as access to lecture notes or permission to record lectures for later review. Using assistive technology, such as speech-to-text software, can also be beneficial.

- **Tutoring and academic support**: Seek out tutoring or additional academic support to help manage difficult subjects and keep up with coursework.

2. Fatigue and Physical Discomfort

Students with CM may experience fatigue or pain while sitting through long classes or studying for extended periods. The physical demands of school, combined with the mental strain of learning, can exacerbate symptoms.

Strategies for Managing Fatigue and Discomfort:

- **Flexible seating options**: Request seating accommodations that allow for better support, such as adjustable chairs or standing desks. Having the option to move around during class can also help manage physical discomfort.

- **Breaks between classes**: Arrange your schedule to allow for breaks between classes or study sessions to rest and manage symptoms. If necessary, consider a reduced course load to avoid burnout.

- **Physical education (PE) modifications**: If participating in physical education or sports is too strenuous, request modifications or exemptions from certain activities. Schools can provide alternative forms of exercise that are safer for students with CM.

3. Attendance and Participation

Just as in the workplace, students with CM may struggle with attendance due to flare-ups of symptoms, medical appointments, or recovery from treatments. Missing school can result in falling behind academically, which can be stressful for students and their families.

Strategies for Managing Attendance Challenges:

- **Individualized Education Plan (IEP)**: For children and teens, an IEP can provide a formalized plan for accommodations and modifications in the classroom, ensuring that the student receives the necessary support. This may include flexible attendance policies, additional time for assignments, and access to specialized services like occupational therapy.

- **Homebound instruction**: In cases where attending school is not feasible for an extended period, students may qualify for homebound instruction, where a teacher provides lessons at home or virtually.

- **Online learning options**: For older students, online courses or distance learning programs may offer the flexibility needed to manage symptoms while continuing their education.

4. Social and Emotional Challenges

Living with CM can be isolating, especially for children and teens who may feel different from their peers due to their symptoms or the need for accommodations. Social anxiety and depression are common in students with chronic illnesses, particularly when their condition impacts their ability to participate in extracurricular activities or social events.

Strategies for Managing Social and Emotional Challenges:

- **Peer support groups**: Encourage participation in support groups or clubs where students can meet others who understand their challenges. Many schools have disability support groups or online communities where students with chronic conditions can connect and share experiences.

- **Counseling services**: Many schools offer counseling services for students dealing with chronic illnesses. A school counselor or therapist can help students manage anxiety, build coping skills, and navigate social challenges.

- **Open communication with teachers**: Developing a strong relationship with teachers and school staff can make it easier for students to advocate for themselves and feel supported. Teachers who understand the impact of CM on a student's daily life can be more flexible and accommodating when necessary.

Navigating Accommodations and Legal Rights

For both workers and students with Chiari Malformation, understanding legal rights and how to advocate for accommodations is essential to maintaining well-being in their respective environments. The Americans with Disabilities Act (ADA) and the Individuals with Disabilities Education Act (IDEA) protect individuals with disabilities, including those with CM, from discrimination and ensure access to reasonable accommodations.

Key Protections for Workers:

- **Reasonable accommodations**: Under the ADA, employers are required to provide reasonable accommodations to employees with disabilities, as long as it does not cause undue hardship to the employer. This can include flexible work schedules, adjustments to workstations, or modified job duties.

- **Job protection**: Employees with chronic illnesses are also protected from discrimination based on their medical condition. If an employee discloses their diagnosis, employers must maintain confidentiality and cannot use the condition as grounds for termination or denial of promotions.

Key Protections for Students:

- **Individualized Education Plans (IEPs) and 504 Plans**: These plans outline the specific accommodations and modifications needed to support students with disabilities in public schools. IEPs are legally binding documents that ensure students receive the services they need to succeed academically.

- **Higher education**: Colleges and universities are also required to provide reasonable accommodations under the ADA. This may include extended testing time, priority registration, or housing modifications for students with medical needs.

By understanding the specific challenges that Chiari Malformation presents in both the workplace and educational settings, individuals with CM and their families can better advocate for themselves and seek out the support and accommodations they need to thrive.

10 Mental Health

Living with Chiari Malformation (CM) can present not only physical challenges but emotional and mental ones as well. For many patients, the unpredictable symptoms, chronic pain, and limitations imposed by the condition can lead to feelings of frustration, depression, anxiety, and isolation. Understanding and addressing the mental health impact of CM is crucial to overall well-being and quality of life.

The Emotional Toll of Living with CM

Chiari Malformation affects each person differently, but for many, the condition comes with daily physical symptoms that disrupt normal activities, including work, social life, and self-care. When managing chronic pain, dizziness, fatigue, or neurological symptoms, it is natural to feel a sense of loss or helplessness. This can lead to:

- **Depression:** Living with chronic pain and limitations often results in feelings of sadness, hopelessness, and despair. The uncertainty about symptoms and treatment outcomes can exacerbate these feelings.

- **Anxiety:** The unpredictability of CM symptoms can lead to heightened anxiety, as patients may constantly worry about flare-ups or worsening of their condition.

Additionally, medical procedures, like surgery, bring their own sets of anxieties related to recovery and future health.

- **Isolation:** Physical limitations or pain can make it difficult to engage in social activities, leading to a sense of loneliness. People with CM may feel disconnected from friends, family, and the world around them, as they might struggle to explain their condition or feel like others do not understand what they are going through.

- **Frustration and Anger:** The inability to do things that were once easy, like going for a walk, lifting objects, or even maintaining a regular work schedule, can lead to frustration and anger. This can be particularly difficult to process when symptoms fluctuate or appear suddenly.

Recognizing the Signs of Mental Health Struggles

While feeling sad or anxious from time to time is a normal part of life, it is important to recognize when these feelings become persistent and overwhelming. The following signs might indicate a need for professional mental health support:

- **Persistent sadness or hopelessness** that lasts for more than two weeks.

- **Increased irritability** or anger outbursts that seem out of proportion to the situation.

- **Chronic anxiety** or panic attacks that interfere with daily life.

- **Withdrawal from social activities** or a lack of interest in things that once brought joy.

- **Fatigue** or difficulty sleeping, even when physical symptoms are under control.

- **Thoughts of self-harm** or suicide.

If you experience any of these symptoms, it is essential to seek professional help. Mental health care is as important as physical care, and addressing these issues early can prevent further emotional distress.

Coping Strategies for Emotional Well-Being

Managing the emotional and mental health impact of CM requires both personal and professional support. Here are some strategies to help cope with the emotional toll of chronic illness:

1. Acknowledge Your Feelings

- It is normal to feel a range of emotions when living with CM, from sadness to frustration. Rather than trying to push these feelings away, acknowledging them can help you work through them more effectively. Journaling or talking with a trusted friend can be a helpful outlet for processing emotions.

2. Seek Social Support

- Surrounding yourself with a supportive network of family, friends, or fellow CM patients can provide a much-needed sense of community. Sharing your experiences with others who understand your struggles can alleviate feelings of isolation and offer emotional comfort.

- Support groups, both in-person and online, can be especially valuable. Many patients find solace in connecting with others who are dealing with the same challenges. These groups provide a safe space to share coping strategies, seek advice, and receive emotional support.

3. Practice Mindfulness and Relaxation Techniques

- Stress can exacerbate both physical symptoms and emotional distress. Mindfulness practices, such as meditation, deep breathing exercises, or progressive muscle relaxation, can help you stay grounded and manage anxiety.

- Yoga and gentle stretching exercises can improve both physical and emotional well-being. These activities not only promote relaxation but also help with body awareness and reducing muscle tension.

4. Create a Routine

- Chronic illness can make life feel unpredictable, but creating a daily routine helps bring structure and control to your day. Whether it's a morning walk, journaling, or setting aside time for meditation, having consistent activities helps maintain mental stability.

- Keeping a daily schedule can also help with sleep patterns, which are often disrupted by chronic pain or stress.

5. Focus on What You Can Control

- Chronic illness often brings a sense of loss, as you might feel like you no longer have control over your body or life. To combat this, focus on what you can control, such as managing your symptoms, eating a healthy diet, or taking steps to reduce stress.

- Setting small, achievable goals—such as walking a short distance, reading a book, or completing a creative project—can help you regain a sense of accomplishment and purpose.

6. Cognitive Behavioral Therapy (CBT)

- Cognitive Behavioral Therapy is a highly effective form of mental health treatment for people living with chronic illnesses. CBT helps you identify negative thought patterns, such as feeling hopeless or overwhelmed, and teaches you to reframe those thoughts into more positive, manageable perspectives.

- Working with a therapist trained in CBT can help you develop coping mechanisms and change the way you think about your illness, which can improve emotional resilience.

Seeking Professional Mental Health Support

Professional help is a critical part of managing the mental health impact of CM. Whether you are experiencing depression, anxiety, or another emotional difficulty, there are various forms of mental health care available:

1. Therapy

- Individual therapy can be beneficial in helping you navigate the emotional challenges of CM. A therapist can offer a safe space to discuss your feelings and develop coping strategies.

- Group therapy is another option, especially for those who feel isolated. It allows you to connect with others who may share similar experiences, offering mutual support and understanding.

2. Medication

- In some cases, medications like antidepressants or anti-anxiety drugs may be helpful in managing the mental health impact of CM. Always work closely with your healthcare provider to determine the best course of action, especially when balancing mental health treatment with medications for CM symptoms.

3. Integrating Mental Health into Your Care Team

- CM treatment often involves a team of specialists, including neurologists, neurosurgeons, and pain management doctors. Including a mental health professional, such as a psychologist or psychiatrist, as part of this team can help ensure that both your physical and mental health needs are addressed.

- Some hospitals and specialized clinics offer integrated care for patients with chronic illnesses, meaning they include mental health support as part of the overall treatment plan.

The Role of Self-Compassion

When managing CM, it is easy to become frustrated with your body or blame yourself for limitations you face. However, practicing self-compassion is essential for maintaining emotional well-being. This means treating yourself with kindness and understanding, rather than criticism, when you face difficulties.

Remember that CM is a condition beyond your control. Being kind to yourself—whether by taking breaks, allowing yourself time to rest, or acknowledging the strength it takes to manage your illness—can reduce feelings of guilt or frustration.

Finding Hope in the Journey

Although CM is a lifelong condition, it is important to recognize that emotional and mental health challenges do not have to define your experience. With proper support, both from loved ones and professionals, you can learn to manage the emotional toll and live a fulfilling life despite the limitations of CM.

Every person's journey with CM is unique, and while there are no one-size-fits-all solutions, taking active steps to support your mental health can significantly improve your overall quality of life. Embrace your emotions, seek help when needed, and remember that you are not alone in facing this condition. There is strength in community, hope in progress, and resilience in the human spirit.

11. Controversies in Chiari

Chiari malformation type I (CMI) presents unique challenges in diagnosis, treatment, and management, leading to several controversies among healthcare professionals [4]. While advances in medical imaging have made it easier to detect this condition, its complex symptomatology and variable outcomes make its management difficult. This chapter explores some of the key controversies surrounding CMI, including overdiagnosis, surgical management, and the debate over the best techniques for treating this complex condition.

Diagnosis Dilemma: Incidental Findings vs. Symptomatic Cases

One of the most significant controversies surrounding Chiari malformation type I is the frequency with which it is diagnosed incidentally. Advances in MRI technology have allowed doctors to identify CMI in patients who undergo imaging for unrelated symptoms, such as neck pain or headaches. In many of these cases, the patients may not exhibit classic symptoms of CMI, but their MRIs reveal cerebellar tonsillar herniation extending 3-5 mm below the foramen magnum, raising questions about the clinical significance of these findings.

Many experts argue that treating CMI based solely on radiographic evidence, without considering the patient's symptoms, can lead to overdiagnosis and unnecessary surgeries. Some patients with incidental findings may never experience symptoms related to CMI, while others with minimal herniation may have significant symptoms, such as severe headaches, balance problems, or neurological deficits. This makes it difficult to establish clear diagnostic criteria that apply universally.

Patient Story: Overdiagnosis and Unnecessary Surgery

Sophia, a 35-year-old woman, began experiencing neck pain and occasional headaches. After undergoing an MRI to investigate her symptoms, she was diagnosed with CMI despite having no other neurological symptoms. Her physician recommended surgery, stating that her cerebellar tonsils had herniated 4 mm below the foramen magnum. Unsure of the diagnosis, Sophia sought a second opinion from a Chiari specialist, who concluded that her symptoms were more likely due to cervical muscle strain than CMI. With physical therapy and non-invasive treatments, her symptoms improved, and she avoided unnecessary surgery.

This story illustrates the challenges of distinguishing incidental CMI findings from truly symptomatic cases. It highlights the importance of a careful clinical evaluation, where both imaging results and patient symptoms are considered before making treatment decisions.

Surgical Indications: When Is Surgery Necessary?

The decision to perform surgery for Chiari malformation type I remains one of the most debated aspects of its management. Surgery, typically a suboccipital craniectomy, is performed to decompress the foramen magnum and improve cerebrospinal fluid (CSF) flow. While some patients benefit greatly from this procedure, others experience little to no improvement, leading to questions about when surgery is truly necessary.

Many surgeons recommend surgery for patients who have clear evidence of CSF flow obstruction on cine MRI and those experiencing progressive neurological symptoms, such as syringomyelia (a condition in which a cyst forms within the spinal cord). However, some surgeons have been criticized for performing surgery on asymptomatic patients or those without definitive evidence of CSF obstruction, potentially subjecting patients to unnecessary risks.

The controversy lies in the lack of standardized guidelines for determining which patients should undergo surgery and which should be monitored conservatively. Some surgeons advocate for a more conservative approach, reserving surgery for those with clear symptoms and diagnostic evidence of CSF flow disruption. Others argue that early intervention can prevent long-term neurological damage, particularly in patients with syringomyelia.

Patient Story: Delayed Surgery and Neurological Decline

James, a 42-year-old man, was diagnosed with CMI after experiencing worsening balance problems, weakness in his legs, and frequent headaches. His MRI revealed a 7 mm herniation of the cerebellar tonsils, but his doctor recommended a "wait-and-see" approach since his symptoms were mild at the time. Over the next two years, James's symptoms progressed, and he developed syringomyelia. By the time he underwent surgery, his condition had worsened significantly, and while the surgery helped alleviate some of his symptoms, he never fully regained his previous level of function.

James's story highlights the potential risks of delaying surgery for patients with symptomatic CMI. While a conservative approach may be appropriate in some cases, for patients with progressive symptoms or associated conditions like syringomyelia, timely surgical intervention may prevent long-term damage.

Variability in Surgical Techniques: Which Is Best?

Even when surgery is deemed necessary, there is no consensus on the best surgical technique for treating CMI. The two most common procedures are suboccipital craniectomy, which involves removing a small portion of the skull to relieve pressure, and duroplasty, which involves opening the dura (the protective covering of the brain) and placing a graft to further expand the space around the cerebellum. Other variations include whether or not to resect part of the cerebellar tonsils and whether to open the arachnoid membrane.

The decision to perform duroplasty or simply remove bone remains controversial. Some studies suggest that adding duroplasty improves CSF flow and reduces the likelihood of reoperation, while others report higher complication rates, such as cerebrospinal fluid leaks or infection, associated with opening the dura. Similarly, tonsillar resection can increase the risk of complications, leading many surgeons to avoid this step unless absolutely necessary.

A key factor influencing these decisions is the patient's specific anatomy and the severity of their CSF obstruction. However, the lack of large, randomized controlled trials comparing different surgical techniques makes it difficult to determine the best approach for each patient.

Patient Story: Complications After Duroplasty

Isabella, a 28-year-old woman, underwent decompression surgery with duroplasty after experiencing debilitating headaches and dizziness due to CMI. Initially, her symptoms improved, but within a few weeks, she developed severe neck pain and swelling at the surgical site. Her surgeon diagnosed her with a cerebrospinal fluid leak, a known complication of duroplasty. Isabella required a second surgery to repair the leak, leading to a prolonged recovery.

While duroplasty is often recommended for patients with significant CSF obstruction, Isabella's story underscores the potential risks associated with this more invasive approach. It highlights the need for individualized decision-making based on the patient's specific anatomy and risk factors.

The Role of Cine MRI: Essential or Optional?

Cine MRI, which shows the flow of CSF in real-time, has become an important tool for diagnosing Chiari malformation and determining the need for surgery. However, its use is not universally accepted, and some doctors question whether cine MRI is necessary for all patients.

Proponents of cine MRI argue that it provides crucial information about CSF flow dynamics, allowing surgeons to tailor their approach and make more informed decisions about the need for surgery. Cine MRI can help identify patients who are at higher risk for syringomyelia and those who may benefit from more aggressive surgical intervention.

On the other hand, some surgeons believe that cine MRI is an expensive and unnecessary test in many cases, especially when the patient's symptoms and anatomy are clear from standard MRI scans. They argue that cine MRI should be reserved for complex or borderline cases where the diagnosis or treatment plan is unclear.

Patient Story: The Role of Cine MRI in Decision-Making

Liam, a 36-year-old man, had been experiencing recurring headaches and neck pain for years. His MRI revealed a 5 mm herniation of the cerebellar tonsils, but his doctor was hesitant to recommend surgery based on the imaging alone. To get a clearer picture of his condition, Liam underwent a cine MRI, which showed significant CSF flow obstruction at the foramen magnum. Based on these findings, his doctor recommended surgery, which successfully relieved his symptoms.

Liam's story demonstrates the value of cine MRI in cases where standard MRI findings are ambiguous or do not correlate with the patient's symptoms. By providing real-time information about CSF flow, cine MRI can help guide treatment decisions and ensure that patients receive the most appropriate care.

Conclusion: Finding the Balance

The controversies surrounding the diagnosis and treatment of Chiari malformation type I reflect the complexity of this condition. With no one-size-fits-all approach, each patient must be evaluated individually, considering both their symptoms and imaging findings. While some cases may require immediate surgical intervention, others may benefit from a more conservative approach. Advances in diagnostic techniques, such as cine MRI, continue to improve our understanding of CMI, but further research is needed to establish standardized guidelines for diagnosis and treatment.

Ultimately, open communication between patients and healthcare providers is essential to navigate these controversies and ensure that each patient receives the most appropriate care for their unique situation.

Chiari malformation type I (CM-1) is a neurological condition where the cerebellar tonsils descend into the spinal canal, potentially causing a range of symptoms, including headaches, neck pain, dizziness, and, in severe cases, neurological deficits. Despite growing research into the condition, the exact causes and best treatment approaches remain somewhat elusive. This chapter explores recent studies on CM-1, focusing on the impact of family history, the underlying pathophysiology, and the role of artificial intelligence (AI) in improving diagnosis and treatment outcomes.

1. Family History and Its Impact on Surgical Outcomes

One of the complexities of CM-1 is the question of whether family history influences the condition's development and treatment outcomes. A 2020 study published in *World Neurosurgery* [1] aimed to investigate this by examining how a family history of CM-1 affects clinical presentation and recovery after surgery in adult patients.

The Purpose of the Study

The primary aim was to determine whether having a family history of CM-1 impacts the symptoms experienced by patients and their surgical outcomes. The researchers focused on whether patients with a family history of CM-1 had different responses to suboccipital decompression surgery—a common procedure for

CM-1 that aims to relieve pressure on the brain and spinal cord by improving cerebrospinal fluid (CSF) flow.

Study Methods

The study reviewed medical data from adult patients treated for CM-1 at Johns Hopkins Medical Institutions between 2006 and 2018. Only patients with cerebellar tonsillar herniation of 3 mm or more were included. The researchers then compared patients with and without a family history of CM-1, looking at their presenting symptoms and post-surgical outcomes.

Key Findings

Among the 233 patients studied, 14 (approximately 6%) had a family history of CM-1. The majority were women, with an average age of 40. The researchers found that symptoms were generally similar between the two groups, but when it came to surgical outcomes, there was a significant difference. Patients with a family history of CM-1 were less likely to experience significant improvements after surgery, particularly in terms of pain relief.

Key Findings on Symptoms and Outcomes:

- **Symptom Similarities**: Both groups had similar symptoms, including headaches, neck pain, and numbness. However, patients with a family history of CM-1 were slightly more likely to experience weakness and cognitive difficulties.

- **Surgical Outcomes**: Of the 150 patients who underwent suboccipital decompression surgery, those with a family history were significantly less likely to experience a favorable outcome, particularly in pain relief.

- **Long-Term Prognosis**: After nearly two years of follow-up, patients with a family history had worse long-term outcomes, especially regarding pain relief.

Why This Matters

These findings suggest that genetic factors may play a role in how CM-1 develops and how patients respond to treatment.

While more research is needed to confirm these results, understanding the influence of family history could help clinicians better predict which patients will benefit from surgery and adjust treatment plans accordingly.

2. Pathophysiology of Chiari Malformation Type I

The exact cause of CM-1 remains uncertain, but it is generally believed to result from underdevelopment of the posterior cranial fossa (PCF), which leads to the herniation of the cerebellar tonsils [2]. This condition can disrupt the normal flow of CSF and cause a range of debilitating symptoms. However, a significant number of people with cerebellar tonsil herniation remain asymptomatic, and researchers are still investigating why this occurs.

Theories Behind Symptomatic CMI

The prevailing theory is that the small PCF in CM-1 patients leads to crowding of the brain structures, which in turn restricts the flow of CSF. This theory is supported by several studies showing that the PCF is smaller in CM-1 patients than in individuals without the condition. However, this theory does not explain why some people with herniation remain symptom-free, nor does it account for cases where symptom severity does not correlate with the degree of herniation.

Alternative Theories

Several alternative theories have been proposed to explain the variability in symptom severity:

- **Tethered Cord Hypothesis**: This theory suggests that tension on the spinal cord caused by a tight filum terminale may lead to CM-1 symptoms. However, there is limited evidence to support this hypothesis.

- **Instability in the Craniocervical Joints**: Another theory suggests that instability in the atlanto-axial (AA) and atlanto-occipital (AO) joints could contribute to CM-1 symptoms. Proponents argue that the cerebellar tonsils herniate as a protective response to mechanical instability. While this theory has shown some promise in explaining symptom development in certain patients, it does not account for the presence of asymptomatic herniation.

Craniocervical Abnormalities and Symptom Development

A more comprehensive hypothesis suggests that CM-1 symptoms result from a combination of anatomical abnormalities at the craniocervical junction, leading to tonsillar herniation and reduced cervical compliance. In this theory, even subclinical instability in the AA and AO joints could cause muscles in the region to work harder to maintain head and neck stability, leading to mechanical overload of the myodural bridge complex (MDBC). Over time, this overload could stiffen the dura mater, further reducing the spinal canal's compliance and exacerbating symptoms.

Microstructural Damage and Symptom Onset

As intracranial pressure increases and compliance decreases, the brainstem, cerebellum, and upper spinal cord experience greater motion and strain. This mechanical stress can cause microstructural damage to neural tissues, leading to common CM-1 symptoms such as dizziness, balance problems, and cognitive dysfunction. Advanced imaging techniques have shown that symptomatic CM-1 patients exhibit significantly higher levels of tissue motion and strain compared to healthy individuals.

The Role of Physical Trauma

Physical trauma can also trigger symptom onset in CM-1 patients. Many individuals report the sudden appearance of symptoms following events like car accidents or falls. Activities that increase intracranial pressure, such as heavy lifting or strenuous exercise, may also lead to symptom development. It is possible that trauma exacerbates pre-existing anatomical abnormalities, causing sudden mechanical failure of the MDBC or other structures at the craniocervical junction.

3. Artificial Intelligence in Diagnosing CM-1

Artificial intelligence (AI), particularly deep learning models like convolutional neural networks (CNNs), is an emerging tool in medical imaging that has the potential to improve the diagnosis of complex conditions such as CM-1. CNNs excel at recognizing patterns in medical images, and researchers have begun applying this technology to diagnose CM-1 based on MRI scans [3].

Deep Learning Models in CM-1 Diagnosis

In a recent study, researchers applied two CNN models, ResNet50 and VGG19, to MRI images from CM-1 patients and a control group with normal brain MRIs. The goal was to assess the models' ability to accurately diagnose CM-1. Both models were trained using pre-processed MRI images, which were standardized to ensure consistency. The training process involved 1,000 iterations, and the models were fine-tuned to recognize patterns specific to CM-1 diagnosis.

Results and Performance

Both the ResNet50 and VGG19 models demonstrated high sensitivity and specificity in diagnosing CM-1. The best-performing model, VGG19, achieved a sensitivity of 97.1% and a specificity of 97.4%, indicating strong potential for using AI in diagnosing CM-1. The use of data augmentation—introducing variations like zooming, shifting, and rotating the images—improved the models' accuracy by simulating diverse anatomical presentations.

Limitations and Future Directions

While the study produced promising results, it was limited by its small dataset of 212 participants. Additionally, only T1 sagittal FLAIR MRI sequences were used, which may not capture as much detail as other MRI sequences like T2. Despite these limitations, the study represents a significant step toward developing AI-assisted diagnostic tools for CM-1. Future research could expand on these findings by incorporating post-operative imaging and clinical data to create more comprehensive diagnostic tools.

Conclusion

Chiari malformation type I remains a complex and often poorly understood condition. Recent research into the impact of family history, the underlying pathophysiology, and the potential of artificial intelligence offers new insights into how the condition develops and how it can be diagnosed and treated. Studies suggest that genetic factors may influence surgical outcomes, while advanced imaging techniques provide clues about how physical trauma and mechanical stress contribute to symptom development. AI holds promise as a diagnostic tool that could improve accuracy and efficiency in identifying CM-1 cases. As research continues, these developments may lead to more personalized and effective treatments, improving outcomes for patients with CM-1.

Chiari malformation is a condition that can bring many challenges and uncertainties, especially during the early stages of diagnosis, treatment, and recovery. However, looking ahead, there is often reason for hope. As research progresses, treatments become more refined, and awareness grows, individuals living with Chiari malformation have a greater chance of leading fulfilling and successful lives.

In this chapter, we will explore the future outlook for those diagnosed with Chiari malformation, the advancements in treatment, and the support systems that help individuals thrive. We'll also look at Pat's story as an example of how it is possible to overcome the challenges and live a full life.

Progress in Research and Treatment

One of the most promising aspects of the future for Chiari malformation patients is the continuous advancements in medical research and treatment options. Researchers and doctors are constantly working to better understand the condition, its causes, and the most effective ways to treat it. Surgical techniques continue to improve, offering better outcomes and quicker recoveries for those who undergo decompression surgery or other necessary interventions.

Innovations in imaging technology, such as advanced MRI

techniques, allow for more accurate diagnoses, which can lead to earlier treatment and a reduction in the long-term impact of the condition. Additionally, scientists are investigating the genetic components of Chiari malformation to better understand who is at risk and how to prevent complications before they arise.

As these advancements unfold, patients will likely benefit from more personalized treatments that cater to their specific anatomy and needs, allowing for more effective and less invasive interventions. The ongoing research offers hope that, in the near future, managing Chiari malformation will become even easier, reducing the fear and uncertainty that often accompany a diagnosis.

Improved Quality of Life

Living with Chiari malformation does not have to mean a life defined by pain and limitations. With the right treatment and support system, many individuals go on to lead lives full of joy, success, and fulfillment. Whether through lifestyle adjustments, pain management techniques, or surgical intervention, those with Chiari can adapt to their condition and find ways to thrive.

One of the key elements to living well with Chiari malformation is learning how to manage symptoms in a way that minimizes their impact on daily life. Many people find that working closely with a neurologist, physical therapist, and other healthcare professionals can help them develop a personalized plan that keeps symptoms under control.

For some, managing Chiari involves making adjustments to daily routines, such as incorporating rest periods, practicing mindfulness or meditation to manage stress, and avoiding activities that could exacerbate symptoms. Others may need more specific interventions, such as medications to manage pain or physical therapy to improve balance and strength.

In either case, individuals with Chiari malformation are not limited by their condition. With the right resources and support, they can continue to pursue their passions, maintain strong relationships, and succeed in their personal and professional lives.

Pat's Journey: A Story of Hope

Pat's story offers a powerful example of what the future can hold for individuals diagnosed with Chiari malformation. Diagnosed at a young age, Pat faced many of the challenges that come with living with the condition—pain, uncertainty, and the difficult decision to undergo surgery. But despite the obstacles, she remained resilient, supported by her family and determined to push through.

After her successful surgery, Pat's recovery process was long, but she never gave up. With her parents' encouragement, her medical team's guidance, and her own strength of will, she gradually returned to her normal activities. While she continued to experience occasional discomfort, Pat learned how to manage her symptoms and was able to resume her education without interruption.

Today, Pat is a successful college student, studying biology with the dream of one day becoming a pediatrician. She has found purpose in her experience with Chiari, using it as inspiration to help others who face medical challenges. Her condition, once a source of pain and fear, has become a motivator for her to make a difference in the world.

Pat's story serves as a testament to the resilience of individuals with Chiari malformation. It shows that while the path may be difficult, there is always hope for a bright future. She continues to inspire others by sharing her experience and demonstrating that Chiari does not have to define one's life.

Looking Ahead: A Positive Outlook

For many individuals living with Chiari malformation, the future is filled with hope and promise. As awareness of the condition grows, so too does the support available to those affected by it. Communities of individuals with Chiari have formed, offering solidarity, advice, and encouragement. These support networks help people feel less isolated and provide them with the resources they need to navigate life with the condition.

Families of those with Chiari malformation can also look ahead with optimism. Advances in pediatric care, early intervention strategies, and tailored educational plans ensure that children diagnosed with Chiari receive the support they need to succeed academically, socially, and emotionally. Schools are becoming more accommodating of students with medical conditions, and families can work with teachers and counselors to ensure their children receive appropriate modifications to their learning environment.

For parents of children with Chiari, the future holds the possibility of watching their children grow up, achieve their goals, and live fulfilling lives. While it can be difficult to accept a Chiari diagnosis, parents can find solace in knowing that with the right medical care and support, their child has every opportunity to thrive.

Hope for the Future

The future for individuals with Chiari malformation is bright, thanks to advances in medical research, the development of new treatments, and the growth of supportive communities. While the journey may be challenging at times, there is every reason to believe that life with Chiari can be rich, fulfilling, and full of possibility.

Doctors, researchers, and advocates continue to push for greater awareness and understanding of the condition, and as a result, more resources are becoming available for those who need them. The days of navigating Chiari malformation in isolation are coming to an end, replaced by a future where patients and families have access to the care and support they need.

Chiari malformation may be a lifelong condition, but it does not have to dictate one's life. With determination, resilience, and the support of loved ones, individuals with Chiari can look ahead with optimism, knowing that their future is full of hope.

14. FAQ

Chiari Malformation (CM) is a complex condition, and it's natural to have many questions. Below are some of the most frequently asked questions (FAQs) about Chiari Malformation, including information about diagnosis, symptoms, treatments, and living with the condition.

1. What is Chiari Malformation?

Chiari Malformation (CM) refers to a structural abnormality in the brain where the cerebellum extends below the foramen magnum (the opening at the base of the skull) into the spinal canal. This condition can interfere with the flow of cerebrospinal fluid (CSF) and may lead to a range of neurological symptoms. The most common form is Chiari Malformation Type I (CM-1).

2. What are the different types of Chiari Malformation?

There are four types of Chiari Malformation:

- **Type I (CM-1)**: The cerebellar tonsils extend into the spinal canal. This is the most common and often diagnosed in adulthood.

- **Type II (CM-2)**: Also known as Arnold-Chiari Malformation, it involves both the cerebellum and brainstem herniating into the spinal canal. CM-2 is usually present at birth.

- **Type III (CM-3)**: A more severe form involving more extensive herniation of the cerebellum and brainstem, often with accompanying spinal defects.

- **Type IV (CM-4)**: Characterized by an underdeveloped or missing cerebellum. This is a rare and severe form.

3. What causes Chiari Malformation?

The exact cause of CM is not entirely understood, but it is thought to result from underdevelopment of the skull during fetal development. In some cases, it may be associated with genetic factors, connective tissue disorders, or other neurological conditions like hydrocephalus or tethered cord syndrome.

4. What are the symptoms of Chiari Malformation?

Symptoms can vary greatly between individuals. Common symptoms include:

- Headaches, particularly in the back of the head and neck

- Neck pain

- Balance problems

- Dizziness or vertigo

- Muscle weakness

- Numbness or tingling in the hands and feet

- Difficulty swallowing

- Sleep apnea In severe cases, it can cause paralysis or impair cognitive function.

5. At what age is Chiari Malformation typically diagnosed?

Chiari Malformation Type I can be diagnosed at any age but is most often detected in adults between the ages of 25 and 45. However, the condition can also be diagnosed in children, especially if symptoms become apparent early in life.

6. How is Chiari Malformation diagnosed?

CM is usually diagnosed through magnetic resonance imaging (MRI). An MRI provides detailed images of the brain and spinal cord, allowing doctors to see the herniation of the cerebellar tonsils and assess CSF flow. In some cases, a cine MRI may be used to visualize the movement of CSF in real-time.

7. Can Chiari Malformation be asymptomatic?

Yes, many people with CM-1 have no symptoms and may never know they have the condition unless it's discovered incidentally during imaging for another issue. These individuals are considered to have an asymptomatic Chiari Malformation.

8. What is the treatment for Chiari Malformation?

Treatment depends on the severity of symptoms. For asymptomatic patients or those with mild symptoms, monitoring with regular check-ups and imaging may be recommended. For patients with more severe symptoms, surgery is the primary treatment option, specifically suboccipital decompression surgery, which aims to relieve pressure at the craniocervical junction and restore normal CSF flow.

9. What is suboccipital decompression surgery?

Suboccipital decompression surgery involves removing a small portion of the skull at the back of the head to create more space for the cerebellum and restore normal CSF flow. In some cases, part of the vertebrae may also be removed, and the dura mater (the membrane covering the brain and spinal cord) may be opened and patched to reduce pressure.

10. How effective is surgery for Chiari Malformation?

Surgery is generally successful in alleviating symptoms for many patients, especially headaches and balance issues. However, it is not a cure, and some patients may continue to experience symptoms after surgery, particularly if they had a more severe form of the condition or complications like syringomyelia.

11. What is syringomyelia, and how is it related to Chiari Malformation?

Syringomyelia is a condition in which a fluid-filled cyst (syrinx) forms within the spinal cord, often due to disrupted CSF flow. It is commonly associated with CM and can lead to symptoms like muscle weakness, stiffness, and paralysis if left untreated. Treating CM can sometimes alleviate or prevent the progression of syringomyelia.

12. Are there any risks associated with surgery for Chiari Malformation?

As with any surgery, there are risks involved. These may include infection, excessive bleeding, CSF leaks, and damage to nearby nerves. In rare cases, patients may develop new or worsening symptoms after surgery. It's important to discuss the potential risks and benefits with your neurosurgeon.

13. What is the prognosis for individuals with Chiari Malformation?

The prognosis for CM varies depending on the severity of the condition and whether it is symptomatic or asymptomatic. Many individuals who undergo successful surgery experience significant symptom relief, but some may continue to have symptoms or experience new complications. In cases where surgery is not needed, patients may live symptom-free lives.

14. Can Chiari Malformation recur after surgery?

In some cases, symptoms may recur after surgery, particularly if scar tissue forms and blocks CSF flow again. Additionally, if the decompression surgery does not sufficiently alleviate pressure, further surgical intervention may be necessary.

15. What is the role of family history in Chiari Malformation?

There is evidence to suggest that CM-1 can run in families, but the exact genetic links are not fully understood. Some studies have shown that individuals with a family history of CM may have worse surgical outcomes or a greater likelihood of developing symptoms, though more research is needed to confirm these findings.

16. Can Chiari Malformation be detected before birth?

Chiari Malformation Type II is often diagnosed during prenatal ultrasounds or shortly after birth due to its association with spina bifida. However, CM-1 is typically not detected in utero and is usually diagnosed later in life, either during childhood or adulthood.

17. What other conditions are commonly associated with Chiari Malformation?

Chiari Malformation is often associated with other neurological or skeletal conditions, including:

- **Hydrocephalus**: A buildup of fluid in the brain

- **Scoliosis**: A curvature of the spine

- **Tethered Cord Syndrome**: A condition in which the spinal cord is abnormally attached, limiting its movement

- **Ehlers-Danlos Syndrome**: A connective tissue disorder that may contribute to joint instability at the craniocervical junction

18. Can lifestyle changes help manage Chiari Malformation symptoms?

While lifestyle changes cannot cure CM, certain modifications may help manage symptoms. Patients are often advised to avoid activities that increase intracranial pressure, such as heavy lifting, straining, or intense physical activity. Staying hydrated, managing stress, and getting adequate rest can also help alleviate some symptoms like headaches and fatigue.

19. Can Chiari Malformation lead to cognitive issues?

In some cases, individuals with CM may experience cognitive symptoms, such as difficulty concentrating, memory problems, or mental fog. These symptoms are usually related to increased intracranial pressure or impaired CSF flow. Cognitive issues are more common in cases where CM is associated with other complications like syringomyelia or hydrocephalus.

20. How does Chiari Malformation affect daily life?

Living with CM can present challenges, particularly for those with severe symptoms. Patients may need to modify their physical activity and be cautious about actions that increase pressure on the brain. Chronic pain, fatigue, and balance issues can impact daily activities and overall quality of life. Support from healthcare professionals, family, and patient support groups can help individuals manage these challenges.

Conclusion

Chiari Malformation (CM) is a complex condition with wide-ranging symptoms and outcomes, but advances in diagnosis and treatment are offering patients better options for managing the disorder. Understanding the basics about CM, including its causes, symptoms, treatment options, and long-term management, is crucial for both patients and their families. Although there is still much to learn, ongoing research and medical innovations provide hope for improved outcomes and quality of life for those affected by CM.

By addressing these frequently asked questions, individuals can gain a clearer picture of what to expect when living with or treating CM. It's important to consult with a healthcare professional for personalized advice, as every case of CM is unique.

14. Beware of Quackery

There are various forms of quackery that claim to cure or significantly alleviate the symptoms of Chiari Malformation (CM) without surgery or other established medical treatments. These "alternative treatments" often lack scientific support, can lead to delayed diagnosis and proper care, and may even cause harm. It's crucial for patients and their families to be aware of these unfounded claims and understand the risks associated with them. Here are some common types of quackery associated with Chiari Malformation:

1. Raw Vegan or Special Diets

The idea that dietary changes alone can cure or reverse structural abnormalities like Chiari Malformation is not based on scientific evidence. While eating a healthy diet can support overall health and well-being, there is no credible research showing that a raw vegan, gluten-free, or any other specific diet can reverse the herniation of the cerebellar tonsils or relieve the pressure on the brain and spinal cord that causes CM symptoms.

Proponents of these diets may argue that reducing inflammation through dietary changes will improve symptoms or claim that toxins in non-vegan or processed foods are to blame for CM. However, Chiari Malformation is a structural condition, not one caused by dietary factors or inflammation alone. While a healthy diet is always beneficial for overall wellness, it cannot cure or reverse Chiari Malformation, and relying on these diets can delay necessary medical treatments such as decompression surgery.

2. Chiropractic Adjustments

Some chiropractors claim that spinal manipulation can cure Chiari Malformation by correcting misalignments in the spine. They may assert that these adjustments will relieve pressure on the brainstem or spinal cord, improving symptoms. However, Chiari Malformation is a congenital or developmental condition related to the anatomy of the skull and brain, not spinal alignment.

In fact, chiropractic manipulations can be dangerous for individuals with Chiari Malformation. The forceful movements involved in spinal adjustments could potentially worsen symptoms or cause injury, particularly if there is compression of the brainstem or cervical spinal cord. There is no evidence to support chiropractic treatments as a cure for Chiari Malformation, and this approach should be avoided.

3. Craniosacral Therapy

Craniosacral therapy involves light touches and manipulations of the skull and spine, with practitioners claiming it can release tension and correct structural imbalances in the cranial bones and spinal column. Some practitioners suggest that craniosacral therapy can help alleviate Chiari Malformation symptoms by restoring the flow of cerebrospinal fluid (CSF).

However, there is no scientific evidence supporting craniosacral therapy as an effective treatment for Chiari Malformation. The notion that gentle manipulations of the skull can alter the position of the cerebellar tonsils or correct the underlying structural issues in CM is not grounded in medical science. As a result, relying on craniosacral therapy can delay proper diagnosis and treatment, including necessary surgical interventions.

4. Herbal Remedies and Supplements

Herbal remedies and dietary supplements are frequently promoted as "natural" solutions for a variety of health conditions, including Chiari Malformation. Some alternative practitioners may claim that certain herbs or supplements can reduce inflammation, improve neurological function, or "rebalance" the body, thus alleviating CM symptoms.

While some supplements, like omega-3 fatty acids or magnesium, may support general health or improve certain symptoms like headaches, there is no evidence that they can cure or reverse the structural abnormalities caused by Chiari Malformation. Relying on herbal remedies instead of seeking medical advice and surgical options can lead to worsening symptoms or complications.

In addition, some supplements may interact with prescription medications or cause side effects, making it important to consult a healthcare professional before starting any new regimen.

5. Homeopathy

Homeopathy is an alternative medicine practice that involves using highly diluted substances to "treat" various ailments. Some homeopaths claim that their treatments can cure Chiari Malformation by addressing underlying imbalances in the body.

There is no scientific evidence to support the efficacy of homeopathy for treating any condition, let alone structural neurological disorders like Chiari Malformation. Homeopathic remedies contain extremely small amounts of active ingredients, often so diluted that no measurable substance remains. The theory behind homeopathy contradicts basic principles of biology and chemistry, and relying on such treatments can prevent patients from receiving the necessary medical care they need.

6. Energy Healing or Reiki

Energy healing practices like Reiki claim to manipulate the body's energy fields to promote healing and alleviate symptoms of various conditions, including Chiari Malformation. Practitioners assert that by channeling energy or balancing the body's energy systems, they can help patients achieve relief from pain or neurological symptoms.

While Reiki and other energy-based therapies may provide relaxation or stress relief, they are not a cure for Chiari Malformation. There is no scientific basis for the idea that energy healing can correct the structural issues involved in CM. Patients should be cautious about relying on such practices, as they could delay critical treatments, such as surgery or medication, that address the actual cause of their symptoms.

7. Detox Programs

Detox programs, which claim to cleanse the body of toxins through fasting, juicing, or the use of supplements, are sometimes promoted as a cure for neurological conditions like Chiari Malformation. Proponents may argue that toxins are contributing to the patient's symptoms and that detoxifying the body will result in symptom improvement or even reversal of the condition.

There is no scientific evidence that detox programs can cure Chiari Malformation or that toxins are involved in the pathophysiology of the condition. Chiari Malformation is a structural abnormality in the brain, not a condition caused by toxin buildup. Detox programs can be harmful, particularly if they involve extreme fasting or unregulated supplements, which can lead to nutrient deficiencies or other health issues.

8. Yoga or Specialized Exercise Regimens

While yoga and other forms of exercise can be beneficial for overall health and symptom management, some alternative practitioners may promote specialized yoga programs or exercise regimens as a cure for Chiari Malformation. They may claim that certain poses or movements can relieve pressure on the brainstem or improve the flow of cerebrospinal fluid.

While exercise can help alleviate some symptoms like muscle stiffness or improve general well-being, it cannot reverse the structural abnormalities of Chiari Malformation. In some cases, certain types of physical activity may even exacerbate symptoms, particularly if they involve movements that increase intracranial pressure. It's important for patients to consult with their healthcare provider before engaging in new exercise programs.

9. Fad Devices and Gadgets

There are numerous devices and gadgets marketed as therapeutic tools for various medical conditions, including Chiari Malformation. These may range from neck braces and spinal alignment devices to electromagnetic pulse gadgets that claim to relieve pain or correct neurological issues.

While some devices, like soft neck braces, may provide temporary relief for neck pain or discomfort, none of these gadgets can cure Chiari Malformation. In fact, relying on unproven devices could delay the pursuit of appropriate medical treatments, such as surgical decompression.

10. Osteopathy and Manipulative Therapy

Osteopathy, which focuses on physical manipulation of the body's muscles and bones, is sometimes promoted as a treatment for Chiari Malformation. Some osteopaths claim that manual therapy can relieve symptoms by addressing structural imbalances in the body.

While osteopathy can be useful for certain musculoskeletal conditions, there is no evidence that it can correct the anatomical abnormalities of Chiari Malformation. Manipulative therapies could pose a risk to CM patients, particularly if they involve forceful adjustments to the spine or neck.

Why Is Quackery Harmful for Chiari Malformation Patients?

The danger in relying on unproven treatments for Chiari

Malformation is twofold: not only do these treatments fail to address the underlying cause of the condition, but they also delay the necessary medical interventions that could prevent further complications or deterioration. Chiari Malformation can progress if left untreated, and symptoms like headaches, balance issues, and neurological deficits can worsen over time.

It's essential for patients and their families to seek evidence-based care from qualified medical professionals, such as neurologists and neurosurgeons, who have experience in treating Chiari Malformation.

Glossary for Medical and Technical Terms

Medical Terms

1.	**Chiari Malformation Type I (CM-1)**: A neurological condition in which the cerebellar tonsils descend below the foramen magnum into the spinal canal. It can cause a variety of symptoms, including headaches, neck pain, dizziness, and, in severe cases, neurological deficits.

2.	**Cerebellar Tonsils**: Structures located at the lower part of the cerebellum. In CM-1, they herniate through the foramen magnum into the spinal canal, potentially disrupting cerebrospinal fluid flow.

3.	**Foramen Magnum**: A large opening at the base of the skull through which the brainstem connects to the spinal cord. In CM-1, cerebellar tonsils herniate through this opening.

4.	**Cerebrospinal Fluid (CSF)**: A clear fluid surrounding the brain and spinal cord, which acts as a cushion and plays a role in nutrient transport and waste removal. Disrupted CSF flow is a key factor in CM-1 symptomatology.

5.	**Posterior Cranial Fossa (PCF)**: A depression in the skull that houses the cerebellum and brainstem. In CM-1 patients, the PCF is often smaller, contributing to the herniation of the cerebellar tonsils.

6. **Suboccipital Decompression Surgery**: A surgical procedure performed on CM-1 patients to relieve pressure by removing part of the skull or vertebrae and improving CSF flow.

7. **Syringomyelia**: A condition often associated with CM-1 in which a fluid-filled cyst (syrinx) forms within the spinal cord. It can lead to progressive neurological damage if left untreated.

8. **Hypoplastic Posterior Cranial Fossa**: An underdeveloped or smaller-than-normal PCF, commonly found in CM-1 patients, which restricts space for the brain structures, potentially leading to tonsillar herniation.

9. **Atlanto-Axial (AA) Joint**: The joint between the first two cervical vertebrae (C1 and C2). Instability in this joint has been proposed as a contributing factor in some cases of CM-1.

10. **Atlanto-Occipital (AO) Joint**: The joint between the base of the skull and the first cervical vertebra. Like the AA joint, instability in this region may be linked to CM-1 symptoms.

11. **Tethered Cord Syndrome**: A neurological disorder in which the spinal cord is abnormally attached within the spinal canal, limiting its movement. It has been proposed as a potential cause of some CM-1 symptoms, though evidence remains limited.

12. **Myodural Bridge Complex (MDBC)**: A structure connecting suboccipital muscles to the dura mater. It is thought to play a role in regulating CSF flow, and its failure may contribute to CM-1 symptoms.

13. **Dura Mater**: The tough outer membrane that surrounds the brain and spinal cord. In CM-1 patients, the dura can become stiff and less compliant, exacerbating

symptoms.

14. **Microstructural Damage**: Refers to damage to the microscopic structures of neural tissue, such as neurons and white matter fibers, often caused by mechanical strain and elevated intracranial pressure in CM-1 patients.

15. **Cervical Compliance**: The ability of the cervical spinal canal to expand and accommodate changes in pressure. Reduced cervical compliance is thought to worsen CM-1 symptoms.

16. **Valsalva Maneuver**: An action involving forceful exhalation against a closed airway, often used in medical tests to assess heart function. In CM-1 patients, this can cause a temporary increase in intracranial pressure, triggering symptoms like headaches.

17. **Hydrocephalus**: A condition characterized by an accumulation of excess cerebrospinal fluid within the brain, often associated with CM-1, leading to increased intracranial pressure.

18. **Cine MRI**: A type of MRI that captures CSF flow in real-time, often used in the evaluation of patients with CM-1 to assess CSF flow disruption caused by tonsillar herniation.

19. **Platybasia**: A flattening of the base of the skull, sometimes seen in patients with CM-1. This skeletal abnormality can contribute to craniocervical junction compression and worsen symptoms.

20. **Filum Terminale**: A fibrous tissue at the end of the spinal cord that anchors it in place. Tension in this structure has been implicated in the tethered cord hypothesis for CM-1.

21. **Craniocervical Junction (CCJ)**: The anatomical region where the skull meets the cervical spine. It is a critical area in CM-1, as abnormalities here can lead

to cerebellar tonsil herniation and symptom development.

Machine Learning and Artificial Intelligence Terms

1.   **Artificial Intelligence (AI)**: A branch of computer science focused on creating systems that can perform tasks that normally require human intelligence, such as learning, pattern recognition, and decision-making.

2.   **Deep Learning**: A subset of AI and machine learning that uses neural networks with many layers to analyze data and extract high-level features. Deep learning models are especially powerful in tasks such as image and speech recognition.

3.   **Machine Learning**: A type of AI that enables systems to learn patterns from data and make decisions or predictions based on that data. In CM-1 research, machine learning is applied to medical imaging for diagnostic purposes.

4.   **Convolutional Neural Networks (CNNs)**: A type of deep learning algorithm particularly well-suited to image recognition tasks. CNNs have been used in the diagnosis of CM-1 by analyzing MRI images to detect cerebellar tonsil herniation.

5.   **Neural Networks**: AI models inspired by the human brain's structure, consisting of interconnected layers of nodes (neurons) that process information. In medical imaging, neural networks are used to learn patterns from complex data.

6.   **ResNet50**: A specific type of deep learning CNN model that contains 50 layers. It is commonly used in medical imaging tasks to identify features in complex datasets, such as detecting abnormalities in MRI scans of CM-1 patients.

7.   **VGG19**: Another deep learning CNN model, consisting of 19 layers, used in image recognition tasks. Like ResNet50, it is applied in CM-1 diagnosis to

identify cerebellar tonsillar herniation in MRI images.

8.   **Training Dataset**: A collection of labeled data (such as MRI images) used to "train" an AI model. The model learns to recognize patterns from this dataset, which it then uses to make predictions on new, unseen data.

9.   **Testing Dataset**: A set of data used to evaluate the performance of a trained AI model. In CM-1 research, testing datasets are made up of MRI images that the model has not seen before, used to measure how well the model can diagnose CM-1.

10.   **Transfer Learning**: A technique where a pre-trained model is adapted to a new task. In CM-1 research, models like ResNet50 and VGG19 are initially trained on large, general image datasets before being fine-tuned on CM-1 MRI images.

11.   **Isotropic Volumes**: MRI data that has been transformed to have equal spatial resolution in all three dimensions (x, y, and z axes). This standardization helps AI models process medical images more accurately.

12.   **Skull Stripping**: A preprocessing technique in medical imaging that removes non-brain tissues (like the skull) from MRI scans to focus on brain structures. In CM-1 research, skull stripping is used to enhance image clarity for AI models.

13.   **Data Augmentation**: A technique used in AI and machine learning to artificially increase the size of a dataset by making small changes to the existing data, such as rotating or zooming in on images. This helps improve the performance of AI models by exposing them to more varied data.

14.   **Cross-Entropy**: A loss function used in training machine learning models. It measures the difference between the predicted outcome and the actual

outcome, helping the model learn from its mistakes.

15. **Cross-Validation**: A method used to assess the performance of a machine learning model. The dataset is divided into several subsets, and the model is trained on some subsets while tested on others, ensuring more reliable and less biased evaluation.

16. **k-Fold Cross-Validation**: A specific type of cross-validation where the dataset is divided into k equal parts. The model is trained k times, each time using a different subset for testing, to improve accuracy and reduce overfitting.

17. **Sensitivity**: In machine learning, sensitivity refers to the model's ability to correctly identify true positive cases. For CM-1 diagnosis, sensitivity measures how well the AI model detects patients who actually have CM-1.

18. **Specificity**: The ability of an AI model to correctly identify true negative cases. In the context of CM-1, specificity refers to the model's accuracy in ruling out individuals who do not have the condition.

19. **Accuracy**: The overall performance of an AI model, defined as the percentage of correctly classified cases (both true positives and true negatives) out of the total number of cases.

20. **Area Under the Curve (AUC)**: A performance metric for classification models, often used with sensitivity and specificity. A high AUC indicates that the model is performing well at distinguishing between different classes (e.g., CM-1 positive vs. CM-1 negative).

Appendix: Resources and Support

Navigating life with Chiari Malformation can feel overwhelming, but there are many resources available to provide support, education, and guidance. This appendix offers a list of trusted organizations, online communities, and other resources to help patients, families, and caregivers find the support they need at every stage of their journey.

1. Chiari & Syringomyelia Foundation (CSF)

- **Website**: www.csfinfo.org

- **Description**: CSF is dedicated to raising awareness, supporting research, and providing education on Chiari Malformation, Syringomyelia, and related disorders. Their website offers a wealth of information, including webinars, research updates, and patient resources.

- **Support**: CSF hosts fundraising events, support groups, and educational conferences across the country.

2. Conquer Chiari

- **Website**: www.conquerchiari.org

- **Description**: Conquer Chiari provides extensive information on Chiari Malformation, including symptoms, diagnosis, treatment options, and surgical outcomes. Their site also offers downloadable brochures and educational materials for patients and doctors alike.

- **Support**: They sponsor research, host annual walks to raise awareness, and offer patient stories for comfort and connection.

3. American Syringomyelia & Chiari Alliance Project (ASAP)

- **Website**: www.asap.org

- **Description**: ASAP focuses on providing education, support, and research funding for both Syringomyelia and Chiari Malformation. Their website features a wide range of educational articles, videos, and a section for frequently asked questions.

- **Support**: ASAP offers an active online support group and regional chapters to connect patients and families.

4. The Chiari Project

- **Website**: www.chiariproject.org

- **Description**: The Chiari Project is committed to raising awareness and supporting Chiari research. Their site offers news, events, and information on ongoing clinical trials related to Chiari Malformation.

- **Support**: Provides links to specialists, organizes fundraising events, and offers downloadable fact sheets.

5. Social Media Support Groups

- **Facebook Groups**: Search for "Chiari Malformation Support Group," "Chiari Warriors," or "Chiari & Syringomyelia Support" on Facebook.

- **Description**: These groups provide a platform for Chiari patients and families to share their experiences, ask questions, and find emotional support from others going through similar challenges.

6. Rare Disease Day

- **Website:** www.rarediseaseday.org

- **Description:** This global initiative is held annually to raise awareness for rare diseases like Chiari Malformation. It provides a platform for patients to share their stories and advocate for research and resources.

- **Support:** Connects patients and families with local events, advocacy opportunities, and awareness-raising campaigns.

7. The National Institute of Neurological Disorders and Stroke (NINDS)

- **Website:** www.ninds.nih.gov

- **Description:** NINDS offers detailed information on Chiari Malformation, including scientific research updates, treatment options, and potential clinical trials.

- **Support:** Offers links to government resources and research studies for Chiari and related conditions.

8. Chiari Malformation and Syringomyelia Support Group (UK)

- **Website:** www.chiari.co.uk

- **Description:** This UK-based group offers resources for patients, families, and caregivers. The website provides information about Chiari, living with the condition, and support networks in the UK.

- **Support:** Offers patient forums and support groups, as well as advice on navigating the healthcare system.

9. ClinicalTrials.gov

- **Website:** www.clinicaltrials.gov

- **Description**: This government-run database provides up-to-date listings of clinical trials, including studies focused on Chiari Malformation. Patients can search for trials based on location, age, and treatment type.

- **Support**: Patients and families can explore potential new treatments and participate in ongoing research.

10. The Brain and Spine Foundation

- **Website**: www.brainandspine.org.uk

- **Description**: This UK-based charity provides support for those affected by neurological conditions, including Chiari Malformation. The foundation offers resources to help patients manage symptoms and understand treatment options.

- **Support**: Offers a helpline, detailed publications, and opportunities for connecting with others.

11. Mayo Clinic: Chiari Malformation Resource

- **Website**: www.mayoclinic.org

- **Description**: Mayo Clinic's website includes comprehensive information about Chiari Malformation, including symptoms, diagnostic methods, and surgical treatments.

- **Support**: Mayo Clinic offers a wealth of information on best practices for treatment and ongoing care.

12. National Organization for Rare Disorders (NORD)

- **Website**: www.rarediseases.org

- **Description**: NORD offers a detailed overview of Chiari Malformation as part of their commitment to supporting those with rare diseases. The site provides information on treatment, advocacy, and access to resources.

- **Support**: NORD provides networking opportunities for patients and advocates, helping families connect with resources and support networks.

Additional Resources for Coping and Mental Health

13. Headache and Migraine Support Groups

- **Description**: Many patients with Chiari Malformation experience chronic headaches and migraines. Search for groups on Facebook or check out the *Migraine Research Foundation* at www.migraineresearchfoundation.org for support and resources.

14. The Spoon Theory by Christine Miserandino

- **Website**: www.butyoudontlooksick.com

- **Description**: This website offers support for people living with chronic illnesses and includes "The Spoon Theory," a helpful metaphor for explaining the energy limitations that many Chiari patients experience.

15. The Mighty

- **Website**: www.themighty.com

- **Description**: An online community where people share their personal stories about living with chronic illness, including Chiari Malformation. It's a great platform for finding encouragement and advice.

This appendix aims to provide reliable, comprehensive resources to help you on your journey with Chiari Malformation. Whether you are seeking medical advice, emotional support, or a way to connect with others who understand your experience, these organizations and communities are here to help.

References

1. James Feghali, Elizabeth Marinaro, Yangyiran Xie, Yuxi Chen, Sean Li, Judy Huang, Family History in Chiari Malformation Type I: Presentation and Outcome, World Neurosurgery, Volume 142, 2020 Pages e350-e356, ISSN 1878-8750,

2. Rick Labuda, Blaise Simplice Talla Nwotchouang, Alaaddin Ibrahimy, Philip A. Allen, John N. Oshinski, Petra Klinge, Francis Loth, A new hypothesis for the pathophysiology of symptomatic adult Chiari malformation Type I, Medical Hypotheses, Volume 158, 2022, 110740, ISSN 0306-9877, https://doi.org/10.1016/j.mehy.2021.110740.

3. Tanaka, K.W., Russo, C., Liu, S. *et al.* Use of deep learning in the MRI diagnosis of Chiari malformation type I. *Neuroradiology* 64, 1585–1592 (2022). https://doi.org/10.1007/s00234-022-02921-0

4. Baisden J. Controversies in Chiari I malformations. Surg Neurol Int. 2012;3(Suppl 3):S232-7. doi: 10.4103/2152-7806.98580. Epub 2012 Jul 17. PMID: 22905329; PMCID: PMC3422094.

5.

Belinda Snow holds two master's degrees, one in education with extensive graduate studies on special education. With over 30 years of experience writing about health sciences, she has dedicated her career to making complex medical information accessible to a wide audience. Belinda has taught at the university level and has a deep passion for educating and supporting individuals facing medical challenges.

Her interest in Chiari Malformation is personal—she was inspired to write *Conquering Chiari Malformation* after witnessing her friend's journey when her daughter was diagnosed with the condition at a young age. This book is a reflection of Belinda's commitment to empowering patients, parents, and caregivers with the knowledge and tools needed to navigate life with Chiari Malformation.

www.ingramcontent.com/pod-product-compliance
Lightning Source LLC
Chambersburg PA
CBHW071036250726
48653CB00005B/1864